ADVANCES IN

Family Practice Nursing

Editor-in-Chief
Geri C. Reeves, PhD, APRN, FNP-BC

Associate Editors
Sharon L. Holley, DNP, CNM, FACNM

Linda J. Keilman, DNP, GNP-BC, FAANP

Imelda Reyes, DNP, MPH, APRN, CPNP-PC, FNP-BC, FAANP

ELSEVIER

PHILADELPHIA   LONDON   TORONTO   MONTREAL   SYDNEY   TOKYO

Editor: Kerry Holland
Developmental Editor: Nicholas Henderson

Editorial Office:
Elsevier
1600 John F. Kennedy Blvd,
Suite 1800
Philadelphia, PA 19103-2899

International Standard Serial Number: 2589-4722
International Standard Book Number: 978-0-323-79260-8

ADVANCES IN
Family Practice Nursing

Editor-in-Chief

GERI C. REEVES, PhD, APRN, FNP-BC, Associate Professor, Vanderbilt University School of Nursing, Nashville, Tennessee

Associate Editors

SHARON L. HOLLEY, DNP, CNM, FACNM, Chief, Division of Midwifery & Community Health, Associate Professor, Department of OB-Gyn at University of Massachusetts Medical School-Baystate, Baystate Medical Center, Springfield, Massachusetts

LINDA J. KEILMAN, DNP, GNP-BC, FAANP, Associate Professor, Gerontology Population Content Expert, Gerontological Nurse Practitioner, Michigan State University, College of Nursing, East Lansing, Michigan

IMELDA REYES, DNP, MPH, APRN, CPNP-PC, FNP-BC, FAANP, Associate Clinical Professor, Pediatric Primary Care NP Specialty Coordinator, DNP Population Health Track Coordinator, Emory University, Nell Hodgson Woodruff School of Nursing, Atlanta, Georgia

CONTRIBUTORS

MEGAN W. ARBOUR, PhD, CNM, CNE, FACNM, Associate Professor, Frontier Nursing University, Worthington, Ohio

JANET R. BEARDSLEY, DNP, CNM, ANP-C, Winthrop Family Medicine, Winthrop, Maine; MaineGeneral Health

AMY BECKLENBERG, DNP, MSN, APRN, FNP-BC, Assistant Clinical Professor, School of Nursing, Emory University, Atlanta, Georgia

SUSAN BRASHER, PhD, MSN, CPNP-PC, Assistant Professor, Emory University, Nell Hodgson Woodruff School of Nursing, Atlanta, Georgia

SHARON BRONNER, DNP, APRN, GNP-BC, ACHPN, Clinical Services Manager, Optum Care, North Carolina

MARY JANE COOK, PhD, RN, FNP-BC, Assistant Professor Health Programs, Michigan State University College of Nursing, East Lansing, Michigan

WANDA CSAKY, DNP, APRN, FNP-BC, Assistant Clinical Professor, School of Nursing, Emory University, Atlanta, Georgia

SHERRY A. GREENBERG, PhD, RN, GNP-BC, FGSA, FAANP, FAAN, Associate Professor, Seton Hall University College of Nursing, Interprofessional Health Sciences Campus, Nutley, New Jersey; Faculty, Age-Friendly Health Systems Initiative, Institute for Healthcare Improvement, Boston, Massachusetts

MELODEE HARRIS, PhD, RN, FAAN, Assistant Professor, University of Arkansas for Medical Sciences, College of Nursing, Little Rock, Arkansas

MEARA HENLEY, DNP, MSN, RN, CPNP, PMHS, North County Health Services, San Marcos, California

JENNIFER G. HENSLEY, EdD, CNM, WHNP-BC, LCCE, Clinical Professor, Louise Herrington School of Nursing, Baylor University, Dallas, Texas

DENISE SOLTOW HERSHEY, PhD, FNP-BC, Associate Professor, College of Nursing, Michigan State University, East Lansing, Michigan

MIN JEONG JEON, MSN, RN, APRN, CPNP-PC, The George Washington University School of Nursing, Washington. DC

LINDA J. KEILMAN, DNP, GNP-BC, FAANP, Associate Professor, Gerontology Population Content Expert, Gerontological Nurse Practitioner, Michigan State University, College of Nursing, East Lansing, Michigan

JENNIFER KIM, DNP, GNP-BC, GS-C, FNAP, FAANP, Vanderbilt School of Nursing, Nashville, Tennessee

ASHLEY DARCY MAHONEY, PhD, APRN, NNP, FAAN, Associate Professor, Director of Infant Research, The George Washington University School of Nursing, Washington. DC

GINNY MOORE, DNP, WHNP-BC, Associate Professor, WHNP Academic Director, Vanderbilt University School of Nursing, Nashville, Tennessee

ABBY LUCK PARISH, DNP, AGPCNP-BC, GNP-BC, FNAP, Vanderbilt School of Nursing, Nashville, Tennessee

SHAUNNA PARKER, MSN, WHNP-BC, Instructor of Nursing, Vanderbilt University School of Nursing, Nashville, Tennessee

JESSICA L. PECK, DNP, APRN, CPNP-PC, CNE, CNL, FAANP, Clinical Professor, Louise Herrington School of Nursing, Baylor University, Dallas, Texas

MARY LAUREN PFIEFFER, DNP, FNP-BC, CPN, Assistant Professor of Nursing, Vanderbilt University School of Nursing, Nashville, Tennessee

GERI C. REEVES, MSN, PhD, APRN, FNP-BC, Associate Professor of Nursing, Vanderbilt University School of Nursing, Nashville, Tennessee

IMELDA REYES, DNP, MPH, APRN, CPNP-PC, FNP-BC, FAANP, Associate Clinical Professor, Pediatric Primary Care NP Specialty Coordinator, DNP Population Health Track Coordinator, Emory University, Nell Hodgson Woodruff School of Nursing, Atlanta, Georgia

SHELZA RIVAS, DNP, WHNP-BC, AGPCNP-BC, Instructor of Nursing, Vanderbilt University School of Nursing, Nashville, Tennessee

JEANNIE RODRIGUEZ, PhD, RN, APRN, Assistant Professor, Emory University Nell Hodgson Woodruff School of Nursing, Atlanta, Georgia

TONJA M.A. SANTOS, CNM, MSN, Baystate Midwifery Education Program, Baystate Midwifery and Women's Health, Springfield, Massachusetts

DEBBIE SILVERSTEIN, MSN, RN, FNP, DNP Candidate, Emory University Nell Hodgson Woodruff School of Nursing, Atlanta, Georgia

JENNIFER L. STAPEL-WAX, PsyD, Associate Professor, Department of Pediatrics, Emory University, Director, Infant Toddler Community Outreach, Marcus Autism Center, Children's Healthcare of Atlanta, Atlanta, Georgia

MELISSA STEC, DNP, CNM, APRN, FACNM, FAAN, Professor and Associate Dean for Evaluation and Educational Innovation, SUNY Downstate Health Sciences University, Cincinnati, Ohio

TAMMI TANNER, EdD, MSN, CPN, Assistant Clinical Professor, School of Nursing, Emory University, Atlanta, Georgia

IRENE YANG, PhD, RN, Assistant Professor, Emory University Nell Hodgson Woodruff School of Nursing, Atlanta, Georgia

STEFANI ELIZABETH YUDASZ, DNP, WHNP-BC, Instructor of Nursing, Vanderbilt University School of Nursing, Nashville, Tennessee

CAROL CATHLEEN ZIEGLER, MSN, DNP, APRN, NP-C, Professor of Nursing, Vanderbilt University School of Nursing, Nashville, Tennessee

ADVANCES IN
Family Practice Nursing

CONTENTS VOLUME 2 • 2020

The Art of Engaging in Serious Illness Conversations with Older Adults

Sharon Bronner and Linda J. Keilman

The Role of the Primary Care Provider in Work-up and Management of Parkinson Disease

Abby Luck Parish and Jennifer Kim

Irregularly Irregular: Atrial Fibrillation in Primary Care

Mary Jane Cook

Managing Older Adults with Type 2 Diabetes: Clinical Insights and Pearls
Denise Soltow Hershey

Women's Health

Sexual Violence Screening for Women Across the Lifespan
Ginny Moore, Shaunna Parker, Shelza Rivas, and
Stefani Elizabeth Yudasz

Wellness and Disease Self-Management Mobile Health Apps Evaluated by the Mobile Application Rating Scale
Melissa Stec and Megan W. Arbour

Hypertensive Disorders in Pregnancy: Implications for Primary Care
Tonja M.A. Santos

Caring for Women with Circumcision: A Primary Care Perspective
Carol Cathleen Ziegler and Geri Cage Reeves

Insomnia Treatment in the Primary Care Setting
Jennifer G. Hensley and Janet R. Beardsley

Pediatrics

Teens and Vaping: What You Need to Know
Jeannie Rodriguez, Debbie Silverstein, and Irene Yang

Autism Spectrum Disorder in the Primary Care Setting: Importance of Early Diagnosis and Intervention
Susan Brasher and Jennifer L. Stapel-Wax

Human Trafficking in the Clinical Setting: Critical Competencies for Family Nurse Practitioners
Jessica L. Peck

Pediatric Fecal Incontinence Evaluation and Management in Primary Care
Mary Lauren Pfieffer

Screening for and Addressing Food Insecurity in the Management of Childhood Obesity
Amy Becklenberg, Tammi Tanner, Wanda Csaky, Imelda Reyes, Min Jeong Jeon, and Ashley Darcy Mahoney

Addressing Human Papillomavirus Prevention and Vaccine Hesitancy
Meara Henley

ADVANCES IN FAMILY PRACTICE NURSING

PREFACE

Nurse Practitioner Role Expansion

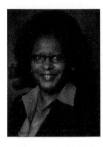 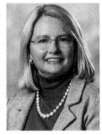 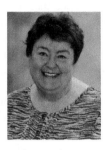 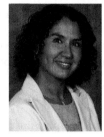

Geri C. Reeves, PhD, APRN, FNP-BC

Sharon L. Holley, DNP, CNM, FACNM

Linda J. Keilman, DNP, GNP-BC, FAANP

Imelda Reyes, DNP, MPH, APRN, CPNP-PC, FNP-BC, FAANP

Editors

Nurse practitioner (NP) numbers have grown from approximately 106,000 in 2004 to 234,000 as of 2017.[1] The US primary care system is a good example of the trend of using more NPs in clinical practice settings.[2] For example, currently there are approximately 2000 primary care retail clinics in the United States. In these clinics, NPs are used almost exclusively to provide basic primary services.[3] In addition, most physician-centric primary care practices have NPs on staff providing care to patients. As NPs continue to grow in numbers, they also continue to gain regulatory support to expand their work roles. Twenty-one states and the District of Columbia currently have awarded NPs some level of ability to practice independently from physicians. This includes the ability to prescribe and see patients without physician supervision.[4] In general, NP role expansion is driven by physician workforce shortages, pressures to expand access to care, patient satisfaction with NP care, and the shift to less expensive value-based reimbursement models of health care delivery.[5–7] More specifically, access issues as a result of the Affordable Care Act's insurance expansion, the aging of the US population, and increased morbidity of the general population in areas such as chronic disease have led to increased demand for health care services, particularly in the workforce arena.[8]

https://doi.org/10.1016/j.yfpn.2020.02.001
2589-420X/20/© 2020 Published by Elsevier Inc.

The impact of role expansion on how NPs experience their work continues to be examined. Literature is quite robust on data demonstrating that NPs and Physician Assistants, as a result of the increased job demands accompanying role expansion, may experience a reduction in perceived levels of internal motivation around their jobs, become frustrated in their ability to feel empowered, and exhibit lower job satisfaction, increased burnout, and greater role strain.[9,10] Alternatively, there is evidence that role expansion not only enriches jobs but also may create a more empowering organizational environment for NPs, which in turn leads to greater feelings of perceived support, self-efficacy, and satisfaction among workers.[11] This empowerment comes from the expanded array of resources, power, and social supports that may accompany the new or expanded roles.[12]

To help support the expanding NP role, in this issue, you will find practice tools and information on prevention and assessment of falls in older adults, extended-spectrum beta-lactamase treatment, serious illness conversations with older adults, Parkinson disease, atrial fibrillation, type 2 diabetes, sexual violence screening, self-management apps, hypertension in pregnancy, caring for women, along with circumcision, insomnia, vaping, autism spectrum disorder, human trafficking, encopresis, childhood obesity, and best practices to address HPV vaccine hesitancy. Resources to support the expansion of NP practice are important for role satisfaction and positively affect patient outcomes. In addition, NPs must engage in self-care behaviors that support work life balance. For example, techniques such as yoga and meditation have been shown to decrease exhaustion, stress, fatigue, and burnout.[13] NP role expansion is a privilege that warrants being responsible to our patients and ourselves. Take time to reflect on how to improve patient outcomes, work-life balance, and in becoming the best you can be–for you!

Geri C. Reeves, PhD, APRN, FNP-BC
Vanderbilt University School of Nursing
461 21st Ave. South
Nashville, TN 37240, USA

E-mail address: geri.reeves@Vanderbilt.Edu

Sharon L. Holley, DNP, CNM, FACNM
Division of Midwifery & Community Health
Department of OB-Gyn at UMMS-Baystate
Baystate Medical Center
689 Chestnut Street
Springfield, MA 01199, USA

E-mail address: Sharon.holley@baystatehealth.org

Linda J. Keilman, DNP, GNP-BC, FAANP
Michigan State University
College of Nursing
1355 Bogue Street
A126 Life Science Building
East Lansing, MI 48824-1317, USA

E-mail address: keilman@msu.edu

Imelda Reyes, DNP, MPH, APRN, CPNP-PC, FNP-BC, FAANP
Emory University
Nell Hodgson Woodruff School of Nursing
1520 Clifton Road, Suite 432
Atlanta, GA 30322, USA

E-mail address: ireyes@emory.edu

References

1 American Association of Nurse Practitioners. NP fact sheet. 2017. Available at: http://www.aanp.org/all-about-nps/np-fact-sheet. Accessed September 20, 2019.

2 Accenture. US retail health clinics to nearly double by 2017 according to Accenture Analysis. 2015. Available at: https://www.accenture.com/us-en/insight-retail-health-clinics. Accessed September 20, 2019.

3 Bryant M. Convenient care, but at what price? The rise in retail clinics. Healthcare Dive. 2016. Available at: http://www.healthcaredive.com/news/convenient-care-but-at-what-price-the-rise-in-retail-health-clinics/415533/. Accessed September 20, 2019.

4 American Association of Nurse Practitioners. State practice environment. 2017. Available at: https://www.aanp.org/legislation-regulation/state-legislation/state-practice environment. Accessed September 20, 2019.

5 Association of American Medical Colleges. Physician shortage and projections. 2016. Available at: https://www.aamc.org/data/workforce/reports/439206/physicianshortageand projections.htm. Accessed September 20, 2019.

6 Centers for Medicare and Medicaid Services. MACRA. 2017. Available at: http://www.cms.gov/medicare/quality-initiatives-patient-assessment-instruments/value-based-programs/macra-mips-and-apms-macra-mips-and-apms.html. Accessed September 20, 2019.

7 Kaiser Family Foundation. Tapping nurse practitioners to meet rising demand for primary care. 2015. Available at: http://kff.org/medicaid/issue-brief/tapping-nurse practitioners-to-meet-rising-demand-for primary-care/. Accessed September 20, 2019.

8 Hoff T, Carabetta S, Collinson G. Satisfaction, burnout, and turnover among nurse practitioners and physician assistants: a review of the empirical literature. Med Care Res Rev 2019;76(1):3–31.

9 Lambert VA, Lambert CE. Literature review of role stress/strain on nurses: an international perspective. Nurs Health Sci 2001;3(3):161–72.

10 Maslach C, Schaufeli WB, Leiter MP. Job burnout. Ann Rev Psychology 2001;52:397–422.

11 Wagner J, Cummings G, Smith DL, et al. The relationship between structural empowerment and psychological empowerment for nurses: a systematic review. J Nurs Manag 2010;18(4):448–62.

12 Laschinger HK, Finegan J. Using empowerment to build trust and respect in the workplace: a strategy for addressing the nursing shortage. Nurs Econ 2005;23(1):6–13.

13 Tarantino B, Earley M, Audia D, et al. Qualitative and quantitative evaluation of a pilot integrative coping and resiliency program for healthcare professionals. Explore 2013;9:44–7.

Linda J. Keilman, DNP, GNP-BC, FAANP
Michigan State University
College of Nursing
1355 Bogue Street
A126 Life Science Building
East Lansing, MI 48824-1317, USA

E-mail address: keilman@msu.edu

Sheila Reyes, DNP, MPH, APRN, FNP-BC, ENP-BC, FAANP
Emory University
Nell Hodgson Woodruff School of Nursing
1520 Clifton Road, Suite 382
Atlanta, GA 30322, USA

Adult/Geriatric

Advances in Family Practice Nursing 2 (2020) 1–9

ADVANCES IN FAMILY PRACTICE NURSING

ELSEVIER
MOSBY

Falls in Older Adults
Prevention and Assessment of Risk in Primary Care

Check for updates

Sherry A. Greenberg, PhD, RN, GNP-BC, FGSA, FAANP, FAAN*

Seton Hall University College of Nursing, Interprofessional Health Sciences Campus, 340 Kingsland Street, Office 4229, Nutley, NJ 07110, USA

Keywords
• Falls • Fall risk • Fall prevention • Fear of falling • Mobility • Older adults
• Primary care

Key points

- Falls, fall risk, fear of falling, and mobility impairment are common among older adults.
- Falls is the leading cause of death from injury in older adults.
- Falls and injury related to falls among older adults is costly.
- Evidence-based tools are available to aid in assessment and management of fall risk in older adults.
- Primary care providers, along with interprofessional team members, have a responsibility to decrease fall risk; promote mobility, function, and quality of life; and help older adults attain person-centered goals.

INTRODUCTION

As the US population continues to age, nurses and interprofessional care providers, at all educational and practice levels, are well-positioned to promote mobility and function, while instituting fall prevention measures and decrease risk of falls for older adults. A fall is defined as "an event which results in a person coming to rest inadvertently on the ground or floor or other lower level, excluding intentional change in position to rest to furniture, wall or other objects" [1](p1). In the United States, one out of three older adults fall yearly.

*Seton Hall University College of Nursing, Interprofessional Health Sciences Campus, 340 Kingsland St., Office 4229, Nutley, NJ 07110. E-mail address: sherry.greenberg@shu.edu

https://doi.org/10.1016/j.yfpn.2019.12.001
2589-420X/20/© 2020 Elsevier Inc. All rights reserved.

One out of five falls cause serious injury, such as fractures or head injury, and falls are the most common cause of traumatic brain injuries [2]. More than 95% of hip fractures are caused by falling and yearly, 3 million older adults are treated in emergency departments for fall-related injuries [2]. Additionally, the cost for falls is high, approximately $50 billion annually [2] with falls the leading cause of death from injury in those 65 years of age and older. Primary care providers (PCPs) have an important obligation to thoroughly assess, manage, and antici-pate issues that may contribute to fall risk and decreased mobility in older adults.

HISTORY

Underreporting of falls is common among older adults, with less than half of older adults notifying their PCP [2]. Hence, it is important for clinicians in pri-mary care settings to obtain a comprehensive history and anticipate possible issues, risks, or concerns that may not be reported. Fall risk increases with the number of risk factors.

Falls assessment should be conducted to guide fall preventive and risk reduc-tion measures (Table 1) [3]. Ask about prescription and over-the-counter medi-cation use noting [3]

- Number, dosage, and frequency of medications
- Psychotropic drugs, benzodiazepines, endocrine, and cardiac drugs
- Medications with drug levels associated with them
- Possible side effects of other medications

Ask if the person has had any past falls or falls in the past year and the cir-cumstances around each fall, noting any potential patterns. It may be helpful to ask if there was any fall near a major holiday or in a season because that may trigger a memory of falling or a near fall. If a fall occurred, discern the following information about the fall:

- Where did the fall happen?
- What time of day did the fall occur?
- Did anything unusual occur just before the fall?
- What was the person who fell doing just before the fall?
- Were there any witnesses present?
- Was dizziness, unsteadiness when standing or walking, or any other symptoms present before the fall?
- How long after any medication was taken did the person fall?
- What footwear was the person wearing and was it in good repair?

Consider how sensory issues (vision, hearing, touch in particular) may impact fall risk. PCPs should ask about any resulting injury from a fall, whether seen by a health care professional or not. Most importantly, find out how the fall occurred. Hearing the person's story helps the PCP and inter-professional team members implement strategies for prevention of future falls.

Falls may also lead to fear of falling. Fear of falling is a psychological barrier to performing and participating in activities [4]. Fear of falling affects older

Table 1
Risk factors

Assess for intrinsic or health-related risk factors	Assess for extrinsic risk factors
Dehydration	Slippery floors
Electrolyte imbalance	Uneven pavement
Orthostatic hypotension	Wet leaves
Infection	Ice
Sensory impairment	Stairs and/or railings in poor condition
Alcohol misuse	Poor lighting
Effects of Parkinson disease	Throw rugs or mats
Balance and/or gait disorders	Clutter in the walking path
Pain	
Stroke	
Arthritis	
Exacerbation of a chronic condition	

adults' decisions about activities they engage in and how physically active they remain. Consequences of fear of falling may include falls, curtailment of activities, disability, immobility, functional dependence, decreased quality of life, anxiety, and injury [5]. The history should also include a holistic assessment of fear of falling. Consider the following questions:

- Is there any concern about falling when conducting activities of daily living, instrumental activities of daily living, or any recreational or social activities?
- Are concerns about falling preventing the individual from doing something they would like to do?
- Is the individual giving up any type of favorite activities related to their falling fear (eg, worship, meals, volunteering, social engagement, trips)?
- What do they think may be done to help overcome that fear or concern?

Answers to these types of questions can help the PCP further assess and consider applicable intervention strategies to reduce fear of falling.

ASSESSMENT/PHYSICAL EXAMINATION

A comprehensive physical assessment should be conducted to assess actual or potential physical-related causes of falls or risk of falls. Although all parts of the physical examination are important, focus should be on the following assessments:

- Vital signs with orthostatic readings (sitting, lying, standing)
- Respiratory, cardiac, peripheral vascular, and neurologic systems
- Musculoskeletal including thorough testing of mobility, gait, balance, and strength
- Cognitive and mental status

Multiple screening tools are available to further assess factors related to risk of falls. Examples of balance and strength tests used in primary care include the 30-Second Chair Stand Test, Berg Balance Test, Functional Reach Test, and Performance-Oriented Mobility Assessment (POMA) [3,6].

The 30-Second Chair Stand Test is a quick assessment of leg strength and endurance [7]. Older adults are asked to cross their arms over their chest while seated in a chair, noting if arms are needed to get up from the chair. Record the number of times the person can fully stand and sit in 30 seconds. For older adults 75 to 79 years old, less than 11 stands in men and 10 stands in women is considered abnormal and indicates increased fall risk [3].

The Berg Balance Test includes 14 items of balance, including timed tandem stance, semitandem stance, and the ability of a person to retrieve an object from the floor. The Berg Balance Test scores less than 40 have been associated with an increased risk of falls [3]. The Functional Reach Test is used to assess balance and postural control. It is conducted using a leveled yardstick secured on a wall at the height of a person's shoulder. The person stands so the top of the shoulder is perpendicular to the yardstick. With the person's fist in line with the yardstick, the person leans forward as far as possible without taking a step or losing balance. Measure the distance of the fist between the starting point (measured when standing straight) and end point (measured when leaning forward) to give the total reach measurement. Inability to reach six or more inches indicates a potential issue and increased fall risk, necessitating further work-up [3].

The POMA is a task-oriented assessment that measures balance, gait, and potential for fall risk. Individuals are timed for the ability to sit and stand from a hard armless chair, maintain standing balance when pulled by an examiner, walk normally, and maneuver obstacles. POMA scores are considered abnormal if there is a one-point deduction from two or more items, or if there is a two-point deduction from a single item [3]. The Falls Efficacy Scale-International, available as a 16-item self-administered long form or seven-item short form, uses a one to four Likert scale and assesses concern about falling during various physical and social activities [8,9]. The higher the score, the increased concern about falling.

MOBILITY ASSESSMENT

The Timed Up & Go test is a commonly used, valid, reliable measure of mobility. The Timed Up & Go measures the time in seconds it takes a person to stand up from a standard arm chair, walk 3 m (10 ft), turn, walk back to the chair, and sit down again while wearing usual footwear and using any usual assistive device [10,11]. Interpretation of a Timed Up & Go score [10] is shown in Table 2.

The importance of mobility assessment and acting on findings is embedded in the Age-Friendly Health System's Model of Care, an initiative of The John A. Hartford Foundation and the Institute of Healthcare Improvement in partnership with the American Hospital Association and the Catholic Health Association of the United States that began in 2017. The aim of the Age-Friendly Health System initiative is to build a social movement so that all care and health care encounters with older adults are age-friendly, meaning care is guided by an essential set of evidence-based practices, causes no harms, and

Table 2
Timed Up & Go Test

Seconds to complete	Mobility rating
<10	Freely mobile
10–19	Mostly independent
20–29	Variable mobility
>29	Impaired mobility

is consistent with what matters to the older adult and their family. The evidence-based set of high-quality care, known as the 4Ms (Fig. 1), addresses (1) what *M*atters to the older adult, considering what is most important to the older adult, family, and caregivers, goals, and preferences; (2) *M*edication, making sure all medications have a clear indication, prescribed at the lowest effective dosage and frequency; (3) *M*entation, assessing and managing cognition, dementia, delirium, and/or depression; and (4) *M*obility, maintaining or improving mobility and function [12,13].

Acting on mobility assessment findings helps to decrease risk of falls, maintain function, and promotes overall safety for older adults. Collaboration with

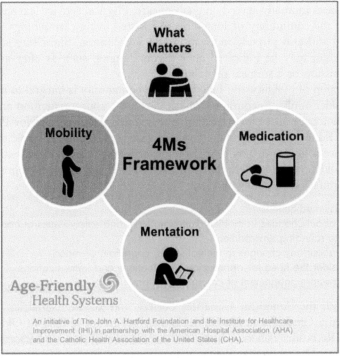

Fig. 1. The 4Ms framework.

interprofessional team members, such as physical and occupational therapists, for more detailed assessment is appropriate, if needed.

LABORATORY AND DIAGNOSTIC TESTING

Consideration of any diagnostic testing to assess potential causes of falls, risk of falls, or injury from falls should be based on results of the history and physical examination. Laboratory tests may include a chemistry panel with fasting glucose and a complete blood count. Diagnostic tests may include radiographs, echocardiograms, brain imaging, or bone density tests, as deemed necessary and appropriate.

DIFFERENTIAL DIAGNOSIS

Differential diagnosis is based on data collected in the history, physical examination, and results of any laboratory and/or diagnostic testing. Conditions that may lead to falls in older adults may be specific in nature or multifactorial including overall generalized weakness, vitamin D deficiency, walking and/or balance issues, medication-related, or any issues related to intrinsic or extrinsic factors.

TREATMENT AND MANAGEMENT

Strengthening and individualized person-centered interventions should be instituted to meet mutually agreed on goals of care. Physical activity (exercise) programs in the community or long-term or assisted living care settings may be beneficial and also provide motivation and socialization. Short stay subacute rehabilitation may be indicated after deconditioning, such as after an acute care admission or a surgical procedure.

Promotion of mobility and function in the community is integral to primary care of older adults. Encouraging physical activity, appropriate food and fluid intake choices, and daily oral health and hygiene are important for PCPs to address. Educating family members and caregivers about fall risk and the importance of reporting any changes in health status cannot be overestimated.

Some older adults may benefit from Tai Chi or similar movement programs. On all primary care follow-up visits

- Assess medications
- Ask about changes in mobility, function, falls, and safety issues at home or in the surrounding environment
- Ask about any changes in mental status, cognition, or mood
- Consider the need for appropriate vaccinations and immunizations
- Follow-up management of chronic conditions

In 2010, the American Geriatrics Society and British Geriatrics Society developed a Clinical Practice Guideline for Prevention of Falls in Older Persons and Recommendations, which may be accessed at https://geriatricscareonline. org/ProductAbstract/updated-american-geriatrics-societybritish-geriatrics-society-clinical-practice-guideline-for-prevention-of-falls-in-older-persons-and-recommendations/CL014 [14]. Common interventions for fall prevention in community-dwelling older adults include the following:

- Deprescribing; discontinuing or decreasing frequency of medications that may contribute to fall risk
- Promoting physical activity and daily routines, especially those related to balance, strength, gait, and mobility
- Managing chronic health conditions, orthostatic hypotension, or sensory impairment issues
- Appropriate supportive footwear
- Consider the need for referral to a specialist (podiatrist, physiatrist)

The CDC: Stopping Elderly Accidents, Deaths & Injuries Older Adult Fall Prevention Program has information for PCPs, such as screening, medication review, fact sheets, functional assessments, and other clinical tools available, and may be accessed at https://www.cdc.gov/steadi/index.html [15]. Training and continuing education, including a video on the pharmacist's role in older adult fall prevention, screening to identify those at risk for a fall, identify modifiable risk factors, and interventions, is available at https://www.cdc.gov/steadi/training.html. Materials for older adults and caregivers to understand more about fall prevention measures may be accessed at https://www.cdc.gov/steadi/patient.html [15].

PCPs may find information provided in the Centers for Medicare & Medicaid Services resources for injuries and falls from immobility useful. These resources are available at https://partnershipforpatients.cms.gov/p4p_resources/tsp-injuriesandfallsfromimmobility/toolinjuriesandfallsfromimmobility.html [16]. Additionally, the National Council on Aging's National Falls Prevention Resource Center has multiple resources about fall prevention available at https://www.ncoa.org/healthy-aging/falls-prevention [17].

PCPs should be aware of evidence-based falls prevention programs available in community settings. Community Aging in Place-Advancing Better Living for Elders, based out of Johns Hopkins School of Nursing, is a 5-month program provided at an older adult's home to decrease fall risk, improve safe mobility, and improve functional status. The team includes a nurse, occupational therapist, and handyman working together to incorporate home improvements and modifications and install assistive devices or equipment to help meet mobility, function, and safety goals and needs [18]. More information is available at https://nursing.jhu.edu/faculty_research/research/projects/capable/index.html.

A Matter of Balance, developed at the Royal Center for Enhancement of Late-Life Function at Boston University, is a group intervention focusing on strategies to increase activity levels and decrease concerns about falling among community-dwelling older adults. Small groups led by a trained facilitator help older adults gain confidence by setting goals to increase activity, view falls as controllable, make changes in the home to decrease fall risk, and physical activity to increase strength and improve balance [19]. More information may be found at https://mainehealth.org/healthy-communities/healthy-aging/matter-of-balance.

IMPLICATIONS FOR ADVANCED PRACTICE NURSING

PCPs have an important role in the comprehensive assessment, management, and planning of care for older adults at risk for falls. Implementation strategies include the following:

- Encourage older adults to remain active and mobile
- Develop a falls risk screening, assessment, and intervention pathway within the electronic health record
- Consider what evidence-based tools may be used to assess fall risk
- Consider how interprofessional team members can complement an initial assessment to address complex fall risk and mobility issues for older adults
- Refer older adults to community-based mobility programs
- Encourage engagement in mobility and fall prevention activities at local senior centers, places of worship, and other community-based programs
- Educate older adults about the importance of mobility, physical activity, and maintaining function
- Educate older adults and caregivers to notify the PCP if any changes in condition (eg, falls, change in mental status, change in functional status) are noted because they may signal an acute medical issue

PCPs, along with interprofessional team members, have a responsibility to decrease fall risk; promote mobility, function, and quality of life; and help older adults attain person-centered goals.

SUMMARY

Falls, fall risk, fear of falling, and mobility impairment are all common issues for older adults and often associated with negative outcomes. Interprofessional teamwork and collaboration is fundamental to the provision of comprehensive, evidence-based care of older adults. PCPs should work with interprofessional team members to assess, manage, and prevent falls while decreasing fall risk, promoting mobility, function, quality of care, quality of life, and helping older adults attain their person-centered goals.

Disclosure

The author has no commercial or financial conflicts of interest or any funding sources to disclose.

References

[1] World Health Organization. World Health Organization global report on falls prevention in older age. 2007. Available at: http://www.who.int/ageing/publications/Falls_prevention7March.pdf, January 31, 2020.
[2] U.S. Centers for Disease Control and Prevention. Important facts about falls. 2017. Available at: https://www.cdc.gov/homeandrecreationalsafety/falls/adultfalls.html, January 31, 2020.
[3] Resnick B. Geriatric nursing review syllabus: a core curriculum in advanced practice geriatric nursing. 6th edition. New York: American Geriatrics Society; 2019.
[4] Bruce DG, Devine A, Prince RL. Recreational physical activity levels in healthy older women: the importance of fear of falling. J Am Geriatr Soc 2002;50(1):84–9.
[5] Brouwer B, Musselman K, Culham E. Physical function and health status among seniors with and without a fear of falling. Gerontology 2004;50(3):135–41.

[6] Reuben DB, Herr KA, Pacala JT, et al. Geriatrics at your fingertips. New York: American Geriatrics Society; 2019.

[7] Assessment 30-Second Chair Stand. Centers for Disease Control and Prevention, National Center for Injury Prevention and Control. Available at: https://www.cdc.gov/steadi/pdf/STEADI-Assessment-30Sec-508.pdf , January 31, 2020.

[8] Kempen G, Yardley L, van Haastregt JCM, et al. The Short FES-I: a shortened version of the Falls Efficacy Scale-International to assess fear of falling. Age Ageing 2008;37(1):45–50.

[9] Yardley L, Beyer N, Hauer K, et al. Development and initial validation of the Falls Efficacy Scale-International (FES-I). Age Ageing 2005;34(6):614–9.

[10] Podsiadlo D, Richardson S. The timed "Up & Go": a test of basic functional mobility for frail elderly persons. J Am Geriatr Soc 1991;39(2):142–8.

[11] TUG Test. Centers for Disease Control and Prevention, National Center for Injury Prevention and Control. Available at: https://www.cdc.gov/steadi/pdf/TUG_test-print.pdf , January 31, 2020.

[12] Institute for Healthcare Improvement. Age-friendly health system. 2019. Available at: http://www.ihi.org/Engage/Initiatives/Age-Friendly-Health-Systems/Pages/default.aspx, January 31, 2020.

[13] Institute for Healthcare Improvement. Age-friendly health systems: guide to using the 4Ms in the care of older adults. Boston, MA: Institute for Healthcare Improvement; 2019.

[14] American Geriatrics Society and British Geriatrics Society. Clinical Practice Guideline for Prevention of Falls in Older Persons and Recommendations. 2010. Available at: https://geriatricscareonline.org/ProductAbstract/updated-american-geriatrics-societybritish-geriatrics-society-clinical-practice-guideline-for-prevention-of-falls-in-older-persons-and-recommendations/CL014, January 31, 2020.

[15] U.S. Centers for Disease Control and Prevention. STEADI: stopping elderly accidents, deaths & injuries. 2019. Available at: https://www.cdc.gov/steadi/index.html, January 31, 2020.

[16] Centers for Medicare & Medicaid Services. Resources: injuries and falls from immobility. 2019. Available at: https://partnershipforpatients.cms.gov/p4p_resources/tsp-injuriesandfallsfromimmobility/toolinjuriesandfallsfromimmobility.html, January 31, 2020.

[17] National Council on Aging, National Falls Prevention Resource Center. Falls prevention. 2019. Available at: https://www.ncoa.org/healthy-aging/falls-prevention, January 31, 2020.

[18] Ruiz S, Snyder LP, Rotondo C, et al. Innovative home visit models associated with reductions in costs, hospitalizations, and emergency department use. Health Aff 2017;36(3):425–32.

[19] Alexander JL, Sartor-Glittenberg C, Bordenave E, et al. Effect of the matter of balance program on balance confidence in older adults. Journal of Gerontopsychology and Geriatric Psychiatry 2015;28(4):183–9.

Advances in Family Practice Nursing 2 (2020) 11–20

ADVANCES IN FAMILY PRACTICE NURSING

Challenges of Treating Extended-Spectrum Beta-Lactamase in Long-Term Care

Melodee Harris, PhD, RN, FAAN

University of Arkansas for Medical Sciences, College of Nursing, 4301 West Markham Street, Slot #529, Little Rock, AR 72205, USA

Keywords

- Extended-spectrum beta-lactamase (ESBL) infection • Beta-lactam
- Gram-negative bacteria • Colonization • Hydrolyze • Enterobacteriaceae
- Carbapenem • Contact isolation

Key points

- Extended-spectrum beta-lactamase (ESBL) infections are a growing national and public health problem.
- The World Health Organization places Enterobacteriaceae into the highest tier and critical priority for research and development of new antibiotics.
- The spread of ESBL infections can be prevented with good hand hygiene and decreased exposure to environmental factors, such as contaminated water.
- Bacteriuria, bacteremia, and colonization are 3 important considerations in the diagnosis, clinical management, and treatment of ESBL infections.
- Delays in identifying ESBL in the laboratory and inadequate empirical treatment of ESBL infections contribute to increased mortality.

EXTENDED-SPECTRUM BETA-LACTAMASE: A HIDDEN DIAGNOSES

The spread of extended-spectrum beta-lactamase (ESBL) infections is a national and global public health problem [1,2]. Multidrug resistance (MDR) occurs when normal flora are genetically altered due to persistent ingestion of large numbers of bacteria through the fecal/oral route and frequent antibiotic use [3,4]. Gram-negative bacteria producing ESBL are one mechanism of resistance to antibiotics [2]. *Escherichia coli* is a common example of gram-

E-mail address: harrismelodee@uams.edu

https://doi.org/10.1016/j.yfpn.2019.12.002

negative microflora that live in the intestines [3,4]. Mutations in normal digestive flora may result in ESBL and multidrug resistance [3–6]. ESBL mutations can occur with just a short course of antibiotics and then live quietly undetected in the intestines for a long time without any clinical symptoms [3,4,7]. Infections can emerge as a urinary tract infection, pneumonia, in a wound, or as bacteremia that is resistant to most antibiotics [2]. The Centers for Disease Control and Prevention (CDC) [8] reports there are 26,000 ESBL drug-resistant infections each year. In particular, older adults with ESBL infections are subjected to higher mortality, higher health care costs, and longer hospital stays [6,9].

ESBL species are gram-negative bacteria [2,10]. Examples of Enterobacteriaceae gram-negative bacteria (Box 1) are *Klebsiella pneumoniae*, *E coli*, *Enterobacter*, *Providencia*, *Proteus*, *Morganella*, and *Serratia*. Gram negative bacteria have a thin cell wall of peptidoglycan [11] and are associated with multi drug resistance [2]. In the United States, *K pneumoniae* and *E coli* ESBL infection rates are trending upward [12]. According to data reported to the CDC in the Antibiotic Resistance Patient Safety Atlas [13], the national rate of ESBL due to *E coli* is 13.4% and 28.5% for *Klebsiella*.

There are more than 500 types of ESBL mutations [10]. Beta-lactamases [5] are enzymes that produce resistance against beta-lactam antibiotics. Beta-lactamases are categorized by the Ambler molecular classification or the Bush-Jacoby-Medeiros functional classification that is based on the ability of the pathogen to hydrolyze antibiotics. ESBL is in Group 2, the largest class of beta-lactamases that inactivates and destroys antibiotics through hydrolysis [2,5,10].

The World Health Organization (WHO) formed a global priority pathogen list (PPL) of bacteria that are resistant to antibiotics [1]. The purpose of the WHO PPL is to determine priorities for researching and discovering new antibiotics. Enterobacteriaceae bacteria are resistant to all or most antibiotics, including cephalosporins and penicillins [10]. The WHO PPL places Enterobacteriaceae into the highest tier and critical priority for research and development of new antibiotics [1]. At the same time, antibiotic stewardship is key for preventing multidrug-resistant infections [12].

RISK FACTORS

There are multiple risk factors for ESBL infections (Table 1). Exposure to ESBL places persons who are immunocompromised at risk for contracting the infection and death [3]. Poor hygiene is a risk factor for ESBL [9]. Other risk factors are older age, recent hospitalization, living in a nursing home, recent surgery, transfer from another facility, an indwelling catheter, and recurrent urinary tract infections [6,9]. Inadequate empirical treatment with antibiotics places older adults at risk for higher mortality [6,9]. However, there may be no presentation of risk factors at all when ESBL infections emerge [9]. Currently, there is no evidence-based standardized risk score to predict ESBL infections [6].

Box 1: Examples of Enterobacteriaceae species

Enterobacter

Escherichia coli

Klebsiella pneumoniae

Morganella

Proteus

Providincea

Serratia

Data from Singleton A, Cluck D. The pharmacists role in treating extended-spectrum beta-lactamase infections. US Pharm 2019;44:HS2-HS6; Schreckenberger P, Rekasius V. Detecting resistance to beta lactams in gram-negative bacilli. Available at: http://www.hardydiagnostics.com/wpcontent/uploads/2016/05/Antibiotic-Resistance.pdf.

TRANSMISSION

ESBL infections are spread through contact with feces or urine [4]. Water can be contaminated with sewage and then ingested into the host through an environmental exposure, such as watering plants [3]. Secretions from the nasal pharynx, urine, or feces are reservoirs for bacteria [3,4]. Food or drink may be contaminated [3,4]. Household pets also can spread ESBL infections [3]. Often bacteria harbor ESBL in asymptomatic patients [4]. Health care providers, family, and those in close contact with the patient unknowingly spread the infection [3,7]. Good hand hygiene is the most important defense for avoiding the spread of ESBL infections [3,7,9].

DIAGNOSIS

ESBL bacteriuria, bacteremia, and colonization are 3 important considerations for diagnosing ESBL. It is common for urine to harbor ESBL infections; however, ESBL may be found in the urine or blood and can provoke an active

Table 1
Extended-spectrum beta-lactamase risk factors: active infection and colonization

ESBL active infection: risk factors	ESBL colonization: risk factors	Active infection and colonization
Age ≥65 years old		Hidden diagnosis!
Recent hospitalization	Comorbidities	Sometimes no risk factors or
Prolonged hospitalization		symptoms!
Severe illness	Severe illness	No universal risk score!
Foreign travel		
Immobilization	Immobilization	
Recent surgery		
Recurrent urinary tract infection		
Nursing home resident		

Data from Refs [3,6,9].

infection that is difficult to control [4,7]. The McGeer's Criteria provide best practices for diagnosing infections [14]. Fever, leukocytosis, acute mental status change from baseline, and acute functional decline should be considered. When bacteremia occurs, the severity of the infection is not related to the severity of the urinary tract infection [15]. ESBL is a billable International Classification of Diseases, 10th Revision code Z16.12 diagnosis [16].

ESBL can be colonized without producing any symptoms [4]. Risk factors for colonization include immobility, comorbidity, and severe illness [9]. One in 10 older adults is colonized with ESBL [9]. Colonization occurs rapidly after antibiotic medications [3]. The oropharynx and stomach are common locations for colonization [3]. The greatest risk associated with colonization is a transition to infection [9]. The intestines may become permeable and leak ESBL into the bloodstream [3]. The course of the infection is further complicated by sepsis [3].

Gram-negative bacteria have a thin cell wall of peptidoglycan [11] and are associated with multidrug resistance that is difficult to detect in the laboratory [10]. There are many ESBL species; however, clinical and laboratory standards guidelines to confirm ESBL only work for *E coli, Klebsiella* spp, and *Proteus mirabilis* [10].

CLINICAL MANAGEMENT

Suspected infections should be treated empirically until the source and sensitivity to antibiotics is determined. The site and severity of infection determines treatment [2]. Because ESBL is resistant to most antibiotics, treatment options are limited [2,12]. ESBL bacteria hydrolyze and inactivate cephalosporin and penicillin antibiotic medications [2]. Carbapenem is the antibiotic medication of choice for treating ESBL infections [2]. Carbapenem improves survival rates [2]. However, carbapenemase strains of ESBL are beginning to show carbapenem resistance [2]. Mechanisms for resistance to carbapenem include *Enterobacter* and *Pseudomonas aeruginosa* [17]. Other possible antibiotics that could be used to treat ESBL include cefepime, piperacillin-tazobactam, nitrofurantoin, levofloxacin, and fosfomycin [2].

The MERINO Trial [18] (Fig. 1) was conducted to determine if piperacillin-tazobactam is an alternative to carbapenem in bloodstream *Klebsiella* and *E coli* ESBL producing infections with ceftriaxone resistance. This international multicenter randomized clinical trial was conducted with participants (n = 391), mainly older adults, from Australia, Canada, Italy, Lebanon, New Zealand, Saudi Arabia, South Africa, Singapore, and Turkey. Participants with bacteremia and ceftriaxone resistance were randomized to receive meropenem or piperacillin-tazobactam. When compared with carbapenems, outcomes showed increased mortality with beta-lactams supplemented with a beta-lactamase inhibitor to treat *Klebsiella* and *E coli* ESBL-producing bloodstream infections. The trial was stopped because of safety monitoring that detected an increased 30-day mortality with piperacillin-tazobactam. So far, carbapenem antibiotics remain the first-line medications for ESBL infections.

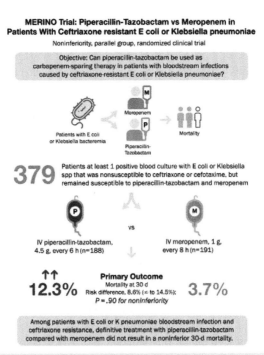

Fig. 1. MERINO trial. (*Courtesy of* Visual Med, Charlotte, NC. visualmed.org *Data from* Harris PNA, Tambyah PA, Lye DCEffect of Piperacillin-Tazobactam vs Meropenem on 30-Day Mortality for Patients with E coli or Klebsiella pneumoniae Bloodstream Infection and Ceftriaxone Resistance: A Randomized Clinical Trial. JAMA. 2018 Sep 11;320(10):984-994. https://doi.org/10.1001/jama.2018.12163.)

One Swedish randomized placebo-controlled single-blinded clinical trial of older adults (n = 80) did not support the use of probiotics to decolonize ESBL-producing Enterobacteriaceae [19]. However, more studies are needed on probiotics and prevention of ESBL colonization [3]. Selective digestive decontamination (SDD) [3] is one method for preventing colonization and antibiotic resistance. SDD is used successfully and thought to decrease mortality in immunocompromised patients in the intensive care unit. The concept is to prophylactically treat the pharynx and intestines for gram-negative bacteria with antibiotics, such as aminoglycosides. International multicenter trials of SDD are needed.

PROGNOSIS

ESBL infections are associated with higher cost, higher mortality, prolonged hospitalizations [9], and overall poor outcomes [12]. The type of ESBL may also determine prognosis. Persons with ESBL *K pneumoniae* (ESBL-KP) are hospitalized more often in the intensive care unit ($P < .001$) [20]. ESBL-KP infections might be more severe compared with *E coli* (ESBL-EC).

Detecting and identifying ESBL in the laboratory is challenging [3]. There is increased mortality due to poor laboratory techniques to identify the type of ESBL [3]. Some laboratories are not set up to test for ESBL. Others only identify *Klebsiella*, *E coli*, and *Proteus mirabilis*. Higher mortality is due to inadequate empirical treatment while determining the specific ESBL infection [9].

Resistance to antibiotics results in limited treatment options and poor outcomes [2,12]. Even when susceptibility to carbapenem antibiotics is determined and there is no resistance, carbapenem antibiotics are expensive [6]. When alternative antibiotics other than carbapenem are used in the treatment of ESBL infection, there are higher mortality rates [6].

DISEASE COMPLICATIONS

Confusion is a well-known complication of urinary tract infections and infections in general that occur in older adults. Older adults have decreased reserve and inability to rid the body of toxins and may respond to infections with hyperactive, hypoactive, or mixed delirium. Confusion clears when the infection is treated.

Another complication of ESBL infection is psychosocial issues. Contact isolation is implemented in nursing homes and hospitals. One retrospective review on early neurologic rehabilitation patients (n = 643) colonized with ESBL showed that the duration of isolation precautions is approximately 19.2 days. Multiple comorbidities, along with contact isolation, contribute to complex trajectory for rehabilitation and tertiary care [21].

The most concerning complication of ESBL infection is increased mortality. A cross-sectional Swedish study (n = 160) showed that inadequate initial empirical treatment with antibiotics is one factor that leads to mortality in severe ESBL infections [9].

EVIDENCE

One in 10 older adults are carriers of ESBL [9]. Models of care are needed to predict ESBL infection or colonization. One systematic review [6] showed a handful of clinical predictor models for ESBL colonization or infection. Predictors included previous antibiotic use, invasive procedures, and transfer from another health care facility. More studies are needed to reliably evaluate ESBL infection risk [6].

A cross-sectional study comparing older adults in the community with those living in a nursing home showed that although rate ESBL infections is trending upward, there is no difference in the rate of ESBL infections in nursing home residents and community-dwelling older adults [9]. Technology using wireless sensors was used in one longitudinal observation study (n = 329) to determine close proximity interactions and the transmission of ESBL in colonized patients [15]. Sensors were worn that measured the distance to an infected participant every 30 seconds over a 4-month time frame. Rectal swabs were collected on a weekly basis. Results showed that ESBL-KP, but not ESBL-EC, was transmitted with close proximity interactions. This supports isolation precautions for colonized ESBL-KP.

CONTROVERSIES

Improved laboratory techniques for rapid confirmation are needed to test for ESBL types other than *Klebsiella* and *E coli* [22]. Rapid confirmation of ESBL will contribute to decreased mortality and promote specific treatment options. Training is needed to detect new species of ESBL. Recommendations from the CDC and laboratory experts in the detection multidrug-resistant bacteria should be more widely disseminated as valuable resources for fighting ESBL infection.

Colonization presents risk for transmission of infection in hospitalized patients [7]. ESBL can colonize silently in patients and health care providers who may unknowingly pass on the infection. At this time, evidence-based practices on how to manage isolation precautions are unknown, especially in nursing homes or in the intensive care units with double-occupancy rooms.

The Search, Destroy, and Restore concept that is used with methicillin-resistant *Staphylococcus aureus* also can be used in gram-negative–producing ESBL bacteria. Cultures from the pharynx or skin are obtained to screen at-risk patients for gram-negative–producing ESBL. Patients are isolated until a definitive result for the specific type of ESBL is identified. After a protocol to decolonize ESBL is implemented, normal flora is restored to the colon. The Search, Destroy, and Restore concept has been successful in reducing ESBL infections. More research is needed on the Search, Destroy, and Restore concept to prevent ESBL infections [3].

One prospective observational study (n = 470) [23] showed that increased infection control resulted in decreased rates of cross-contamination of ESBL colonization in double-occupancy rooms in an intensive care unit. The average duration of clinical isolation on a rehabilitation unit is approximately 20 days [21], which can contribute to depression and decrease quality of life.

Due to clinical isolation precautions for ESBL infection, one retrospective study [21] reviewed medical records to investigate if patients on a rehabilitation unit with ESBL colonization received less therapy than patients without ESBL colonization. Results showed that decreases in independent function were due to comorbid conditions on admission rather than limited therapy due to isolation for ESBL colonization. Although declines in functioning are not associated with decreased therapy in this study, mental health and quality of life related to prolonged isolation should be further investigated.

Although ESBL infections have increased, one cross-sectional comparison study [9] showed no difference between the prevalence of ESBL in nursing homes and community-dwelling older adults. A nursing home is a resident's home. and social withdrawal because of isolation for ESBL infection may be worse than the disease process itself. Any prolonged stay results in detachment from a home environment that can be especially confusing for older adults with cognitive impairment. Further, older adults who are colonized with ESBL may be denied admission to nursing homes, placing them at risk for disparate access to treatment and health care resources. More research is needed on specific ESBL types and patient benefits and disadvantages of clinical isolation protocols for active ESBL infections and colonization.

Methenamine is a 100-year old medication that shows promise for preventing gram-negative lower recurrent urinary tract infections [24]. Methenamine hippurate and methenamine mandelate are available in the United States and are used as maintenance antibiotics. Methenamine is rapidly absorbed by mouth and converts to formaldehyde in the acidic environment in urine. Ascorbic acid can be administered with methenamine to lower urine pH and enhance the effects of the medication. The half-life of methenamine is 3 to 4 hours and is excreted through the kidneys. Contraindications include sensitivity to methenamine, concurrent use with sulfonamides, and a creatinine clearance less than 50 mL/min. The formaldehyde product of methenamine has antiseptic rather than antibiotic properties, making antibiotic resistance unlikely. Overall, methenamine has a good safety profile. Along with good hygiene and hydration, methenamine may be considered as a safe treatment for recurrent urinary tract infections without contributing to multidrug resistance [24].

CLINICAL IMPLICATIONS

Increased morbidity and mortality associated with ESBL infections is on the rise. This silent diagnosis is emerging ahead of research for new antibiotics. The generation of new multidrug-resistant bacteria is trending upward, whereas in adults, the health and quality of life, especially for older adults, is spiraling downward. Education and prevention strategies are key in eliminating the severe consequences of ESBL infections. The WHO supports research for new antibiotics [1]. Given that drug resistance was discovered before the use of penicillin [2], it may be that antibiotics that are used to fight infection actually generate a more complex disease process and no cures for even the simplest infections. Health care providers must use a thoughtful holistic approach, exercise wisdom to master the art and science of medicine, and implement evidence-based practices to guide antibiotic stewardship. Ironically, it may be that lessons learned from the past when there were few antibiotics will actually support a future with fewer antibiotics and obsolete ESBL infections.

Disclosure

M. Harris has no conflict of interest and no disclosures.

References

[1] World Health Organization. Global priority list of antibiotic-resistant bacteria to guide research, discovery, and development of new antibiotics 2019. Available at: https://www.who.int/medicines/publications/WHO-PPL-Short_Summary_25Feb-ET_NM_WHO.pdf.

[2] Singleton A. The pharmacists role in treating extended-spectrum beta-lactamase infections. US Pharm 2019;44:HS2–6.

[3] Carlet J. The gut is the epicentre of antibiotic resistance. Antimicrob Resist Infect Control 2012;39; https://doi.org/10.1186/2047-2994-1-39.

[4] Global Alliance for Infections in Surgery. Antibiotics and antimicrobial resistance. The role of gut microbiota. Available at: https://infectionsinsurgery.org/antibiotics-and-antimicrobial-resistance-the-role-of-gut-microbiota/.

[5] Global Alliance for Infections in Surgery. What are beta/lactamases?. 2019. Available at: https://infectionsinsurgery.org/what-are-beta-lactamases-and-what-are-their-significance-in-antibiotic-drug-resistance/.

[6] Sazlly SM, Wong PL, Sulaiman H, et al. Clinical prediction models for ESBL-Enterobacteriaceae colonization or infection: a systematic review. J Hosp Infect 2019;102:16.

[7] Thaden JT, Fowler VG, Sexton DJ, et al. Increasing incidence of extended-spectrum beta-lactamase producing *Escherichea coli* in community hospitals throughout the Southeastern United States. Infect Control Hosp Epidemiol 2016;37:49–54.

[8] Center for Disease Control and Prevention (CDC), National Center for Emerging and Zoonotic Infectious Diseases (NCEZID), Division of Healthcare Quality Promotion. Antibiotic/antimicrobial resistance (A/AMR). In: Biggest threats data. 2018. Available at: https://www.cdc.gov/drugresistance/biggest_threats.html.

[9] Blom A, Ahl J, Mansson F, et al. The prevalence of ESBL-producing Enterobacteriaceae in a nursing home setting compared with elderly living at home: cross sectional comparison. BMC Infect Dis 2016;111:1430–5.

[10] Neural Academy. Gram positive vs gram negative bacteria. Available at: https://www.youtube.com/watch?v=Didrc3wJ3E8.

[11] McDaniel J, Schweizer M, Crabb V, et al. Incidence of extended-spectrum beta-lactamase *Escherichia coli* and *Klebsiella* infections in the United States: a systematic review. Infect Control Hosp Epidemiol 2017;38:1209–15.

[12] Centers for Disease Control and Prevention. Antibiotic patient safety atlas: antibiotic resistance HAI data. Available at: https://gis.cdc.gov/grasp/PSA/Downloads/AR-Summary.pdf.

[13] Schreckenberger P, Rekasius V. Detecting resistance to beta lactams in gram-negative bacilli. Available at: http://www.hardydiagnostics.com/wpcontent/uploads/2016/05/Antibiotic-Resistance.pdf.

[14] Stone ND, Ashraf MS, Calder J, et al. Surveillance definitions of infections in long-term care facilities: revisiting the McGeer Criteria. Infect Control Hosp Epidemiol 2012;33:965–77.

[15] Duval A, Obadia T, Boelle P-Y, et al. Close proximity interactions support transmission of ESBL-K. pneumoniae but not ESBL-E. coli in healthcare settings. PLoS Comput Biol 2019;15:e1006496.

[16] ICD Codes. ICD-10-CM Code Z16.12. Extended spectrum beta lactamase (ESBL) resistance. Available at: https://icd.codes/icd10cm/Z1612.

[17] Oliphant CM, Eroschenko K. Antibiotic resistance, part 2: gram-negative pathogens. JNP 2015;11:79–83.

[18] Harris PNA, Tambyah PA, Lye DC, et al. Effect of piperacillin-tazobactam vs meropenem on 30-day mortality for patients with *E coli* or *Klebsiella pneumoniae* bloodstream infection and ceftriaxone resistance: a randomized clinical trial. JAMA 2018;320(10):984–94.

[19] Ljungquist O, Kampann C, Resman F, et al. Probiotics for intestinal decolonization of ESBL-producing Enterobacteriaceae: a randomized, placebo-controlled trial. Clin Microbiol Infect 2019; https://doi.org/10.1016/j.cmi.2019.08.019.

[20] Davido B, deTruchis P, Lawrence C, et al. Extended-spectrum beta-lactamase (ESBL)-producing *Escherichia coli* versus *Klebsiella pneumoniae*: does type of germ really matter? Infect Control Hosp Epidemiol 2018;39:1137–8.

[21] Rollnik JD. Outcome of early neurological rehabilitation patients colonized with extended-spectrum beta-lactamase (ESBL) producing bacteria. OJTR 2015;3:1–8.

[22] Thomson KS. Controversies about extended-spectrum and AmpC beta-lactamases. Emerg Infect Dis 2001;7(2):333–6. Available at: wwwnc.cdc.gov/eid/article/7/2/70-0333_article.

[23] Repesse X, Artiguenave M, Paktoris-papines S, et al. Epidemiology of extended-spectrum beta-lactamase-producing Enterobacteriaceae in an intensive care unit with no single rooms. Ann Intensive Care 2017;7:73.
[24] Lo TS, Hammer KDP, Zegarra M, et al. Methenamine: a forgotten drug for preventing recurrent urinary tract infection in a multidrug resistance era. Expert Rev Anti Infect Ther 2014;12(5):549–54.

Advances in Family Practice Nursing 2 (2020) 21–36

ADVANCES IN FAMILY PRACTICE NURSING

The Art of Engaging in Serious Illness Conversations with Older Adults

Sharon Bronner, DNP, APRN, GNP-BC, ACHPN[a],*,
Linda J. Keilman, DNP, MSN, GNP-BC[b]

[a]Optum Care, NC, USA; [b]Michigan State University College of Nursing, 1355 Bogue St, East Lansing, MI 48824, USA

Keywords

- Serious illness • Advance care planning • Directives • Older adults
- Communication • Conversations

Key points

- Aging, dying, and EOL conversations are extremely difficult—emotionally and spiritually.
- Silence is a powerful treasure and allows OAs and families time to process, explore thoughts, and identify their own personal feelings.
- Advance care planning is a lifelong living process that should be created as early as age 18 years and reviewed every year and whenever a change has occurred in one's life.
- Presence, or being with, is a gift.
- The PCP should speak less than 50% of the time during the SIC.

INTRODUCTION

One of the most important concepts Advanced Practice Registered Nurse (APRN) students learn in their graduate education journey is that effective, optimal, meaningful communication is imperative to building healthy relationships with patients across the lifespan. Healthy provider-patient relationships should lead to trust, care, respectful collaboration, and shared mutual decision-making. This respectful process toward decisions aids in determining the best individualized evidence-based (EB) treatment of wellness and disease

*Corresponding author. 928 Parkway Place, Peekskill, NY 10566. E-mail address: sbronner@optum.com

https://doi.org/10.1016/j.yfpn.2019.12.003
2589-420X/20/© 2020 Elsevier Inc. All rights reserved.

management. Mutual respect and sharing of essential health care knowledge and information between provider and patient/family leads to improved adherence to the treatment plan, which leads to better patient outcomes. And when the end is near, it is hoped that transparent, morally sound, and ethical conversations lead to a peaceful death, resulting in less pain and suffering for the patient, their family, and the interdisciplinary team (IDT).

If we are living–we are aging; living on this earth eventually comes to an end. Although health care providers (HCP) cannot prevent death, they can be engaged in compassionate care where EB treatment/management is carried out to prevent the potential untoward aspects of death at the end of life (EOL). Through nonpharmacologic and pharmacologic interventions, the hopes, wishes, and expressed sentiments of the patient can be carried out in fulfillment of their life, and EOL, goals. This is a remarkable opportunity for the APRN to make a difference in the life, and death, of one unique human being who is completing their journey on earth.

Accomplishing a pain and symptom free quality of life (QoL) can only be achieved through intentional listening that leads to artful communication. Therapeutic communication is the solid foundation for everything else that occurs between the patient and the APRN. Even listening becomes a learned skill of intention and purpose; it is more than hearing words, it is about building trust that is enhanced by mutual respect and understanding the tone and emotion that the words and body language convey. Words can deliver pain or hope; it is within the care, warmth, and connectedness demonstrated by the skilled APRN with patients that makes the difference. Because all human beings are unique, every relationship requires work and ongoing motivation to communicate in an individualized manner–to recognize the uniqueness of the person above all voiced symptoms and chief concerns.

According to the Centers for Disease Control and Prevention, health communication is using strategies to inform and influence patient actions and decision making [1]. This definition might make one think all the work is on the HCP, a way to converse with patients that possibly gets them to think the way the HCP thinks they should. Communication is much more than that! Communication should become a conversation; a flow or exchange of words, in more than voice (written, visual, nonverbal). Human beings are constantly communicating–it is a cyclical process of sending and receiving information. Determining *what* is said and *how* it is said is up to the APRN. Although conversations with patients can be simple and straightforward, we also know that health conversations can be emotional, difficult, critical, high-stake, and life-changing. These types of conversations require the HCP to value reflection, honor multiple perspectives, be self-aware [2], have courage, and most of all to have established a solid relationship based on mutual trust and respect with patients and their families. This article focuses on having serious illness conversations (SICs) with older adults (OAs), including the palliative care (PC) option.

OLDER ADULTS AND CHRONIC ILLNESS

Globally, 8.5% (617 million) of the world population is aged 65 years and older [3]. This number is projected to reach 17% (1.6 billion) by 2050 [3]. What should the APRN working with OAs be thinking about related to this age surge? Definitely the need to be prepared to better understand how to care and communicate with the OA and how to have SICs that are meaningful and hopeful. OAs may die from chronic illnesses, such as:

- Diabetes
- Cardiac disease
- Heart failure (HF)
- Cancer
- Chronic liver disease
- Chronic obstructive pulmonary disease (COPD)
- Dementia
- Renal failure
- Peripheral vascular disease
- Multiple systems failure
- Natural causes (Fig. 1) [4]

The more accumulated chronic conditions a person is living with contributes to the complexity of treatment and management. The more symptoms, the more diseases, the closer the individual is to their EOL journey. Chronic illness symptom management and EOL care is challenging in all practice settings, but especially in long-term care (LTC) [5]. In 2006, an estimated 37 million people in the United States were 65 years and older. Projections forecast by 2030, approximately 71.5 million people will be 65 years and older, representing nearly 20% of the total US population [6–9]. Death is inevitable in the life cycle; acknowledging the way an OA can decrease suffering and pain at the EOL is an essential skill for APRNs working with OAs, especially those with comorbid chronic conditions. Nearly 1.8 million deaths occurred in persons aged 65

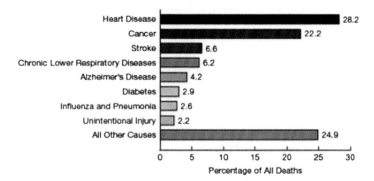

Fig. 1. Causes of death among US adults aged 65 years or older, 2007. (*From* Heron MP. Deaths: Leading causes for 2004. National vital statistics vol 56 no 5. Hyattsville, MD: National Center for Health Statistics. 2007.)

years and over in 2009 [10]. Thirty-two percent of these deaths occurred while the decedent was a hospital inpatient; 27% were in nursing homes or other LTC facility [10]. Currently, approximately 20% of all deaths occur in nursing homes. It has been suggested this number will climb to approximately 40% by 2020 [6]. Fear of an individual dying in a nursing home is a concern with LTC staff. Transferring the dying patient to a hospital, rather than trying to treat the symptom in LTC, is the preference of most nurses. Understanding the importance of SICs can alleviate symptoms through the dying process and beyond for the patient, their family, and the IDT.

Working with OAs is multifaceted and tends to make having good conversations difficult. The lack of a SIC can lead to a death with unnecessary suffering. SIC is an important component of delivering a concise message and honoring the wishes of the patient and their family. Initiating the conversation has been a struggle in the primary care setting (PCS). Asking the question: "would you be surprised if this patient died in 12 months?" [11] has assisted with screening high-risk patients who may be classified with high mortality risk. In a 2019 Dana-Farber Cancer Institute report, "only 1/3 of individuals in their last year of life reported having any conversations and, often, they happen too late in the course of illness to fulfill their most important wishes" [12]. The final year of living with comorbid chronic conditions is generally laden with uncertainty and emotional/spiritual distress when no honest, heartfelt conversations have been explored with the OA. Life does not have to end in this manner—there are options and the art of SICs can be learned!

ADVANCE CARE PLANNING

Life can be unpredictable at any age; an unexpected crisis or illness can occur at any time during a person's lifetime. Although thinking about possibilities or what *might* happen in the future is not easy, it is imperative to look forward to tomorrow as much as to live fully today. If one embraces their independence and values their ability to make decisions for themselves, advance care planning (ACP) is essential. ACP involves learning and thinking proactively about decisions that need to be made during crises that will ensure one's preferences will be carried out by others [13]. A document, an advance directive (AD), is created that specifies an individuals preferences about what they would like medically done (or *not* done) if they are not able to communicate for themselves at the time.

An AD should be created by a competent individual who has the capacity to make decisions for themselves at the time of development. It is important to gain input from loved ones, HCP, family members, friends, faith leaders, or whomever the individual feels are important to them. Legal advice is not required but can always be important in understanding the laws of individual states, because they are all different. A legal representative can also ensure your wishes are carried out when the time comes. When healthy, patients occasionally find the document to be difficult to complete. The HCP can help with some information, such as family history and risk factors. This is an SIC in itself—educating the person about how specific disease states and illnesses are genetically and environmentally caused.

The AD needs to be in writing. There are forms available online—some free and some with cost. A person can also create their own document. It is important to understand that, with any form used, it must comply with the requirements of the state where you live. Five Wishes is an AD written in common language that can help anyone understand the process. It is available electronically, has a small cost, but is comprehensive and thoughtful. The APRN may want to have copies of the document in the PCS to provide to patients when they turn 18 years or when they are your patient. The Five Wishes source is available at https://fivewishes.org/shop/order/product/five-wishes. Some state hospital associations, hospice or palliative care organizations, legal offices, your state representative, or area agencies on aging can also help the individual with guidelines and documents. There truly is no excuse for not having information and forms available in primary care practices. It is the HCP responsibility to regularly ask patients whether they have engaged in ACP or have an AD. It is important to remember there are a variety of names used for the decision-making process so be sure to use some of the common words where you practice.

In the AD, the person needs to designate 1 or 2 individuals (eg, proxy, Durable Power of Attorney for Health Care [legal document], surrogate, designated decision-maker) with whom they have discussed their wishes, preferences, and choices, and who promise to follow the written wishes when, and if, the time comes. This is perhaps one of the most important parts of the process—finding individuals who—even if they do not agree with the decisions—guarantee they will speak on the behalf of the individual. Selection is very important in this component of the living document process. These individuals can be changed at any time. Their signatures need to be witnessed by 2 individuals not related to them or the author of the AD. The author's signature with the date is also needed. On all signatures and dates being entered, copies should be given to the HCP, and individuals who will speak on the person's behalf and anyone else. The document should be reviewed and updated at minimum yearly by the HCP and patient. The HCP needs to make sure the individuals still all agree to their role in the process. Review also needs to occur anytime the health or life circumstances of the individual change. Documents need to be up-to-date and accurate in the primary care office! ACP is an ongoing conversation, which includes reviewing the AD.

Every time the ACP process is completed, an SIC has occurred. Keeping current on state laws regarding EOL is extremely important for the APRN. If, and when, changes occur, it is up to the APRN to bring the ACP process forward at an appointment. The surrogate, health care proxy, or designated decision-maker is often involved in the decision-making process in LTC. The goal is to ensure the OA values, wishes, preferences, and choices are acknowledged during the communication process. The goals of care are crucial to the ACP of the OA.

At present, voluntary ACP is covered as part of the yearly Medicare Wellness visit under Medicare Part B [14]. The APRN will need to check with billing information specialists for their practice because insurance coverage by other than Medicare varies from state to state—even within the type of insurance.

PALLIATIVE CARE

One area of health care that generally does well with SICs is PC, a philosophy of care that enhances the value of care for seriously ill OAs [10,15]. PC begins with the understanding that every patient has his or her own story, relationships, and culture. An SIC combines the dynamic opportunity to hear the OA and family wishes and worries. PC principles and practices can be integrated into any health care setting, delivered by all clinicians, and supported by PC specialists who are part of an IDT with the professional qualifications, education, training, and support needed to deliver optimal patient-centered and family-centered care [16]. PC is a holistic IDT approach to the entire spectrum of care (cultural, environmental, genetic, medical, nursing, psychological, social, spiritual) for all ages, cultures, and races. According to the World Health Organization, PC is "an approach that improves the QoL of patients and their families facing the problems associated with life-threatening illness" [17]. PC goals are "to regard death as part of life and a normal process, neither to hasten nor to delay death, to use a team approach to address the needs of patients and their families, including bereavement." [18].

The principles of PC are presented in Box 1.

Box 1: Principles of palliative care

- Provides relief from pain and other distressing symptoms
- Affirms life and regards dying as a normal process
- Intends neither to hasten nor postpone death
- Integrates the psychological and spiritual aspects of patient care
- Offers a support system to help patients live as actively as possible until death
- Offers a support system to help the family cope during the patients' illness and in their own bereavement
- Uses a team approach to address the needs of patients and their families, including bereavement counseling, if indicated
- Will enhance QoL and may also positively influence the course of illness
- Is applicable early in the course of illness, in conjunction with other therapies that are intended to prolong life, such as chemotherapy or radiation therapy, and includes those investigations needed to better understand and manage distressing clinical complications

From World Health Organization. Cancer. WHO Definition of Palliative Care. Available at: https://www.who.int/cancer/palliative/definition/en/.

PC starts with a comprehensive assessment and highlights patient and family engagement, communication, care coordination, and continuity of care across health care settings. The American Nurses Association states "the aims of nursing actions are to protect, promote and optimize health; prevent illness and injury; alleviate suffering" [19,20]. Goals of care can achieve easing of symptoms, improve quality of life, and support loved ones and caregivers. Frequently, OAs in primary care are unable to make their own decisions about their wishes due to comorbid conditions. ACP requires SICs to have an organized framework [21,22]. Lines of communication must be clear to develop a PC plan. It is important to be honest with the communication delivered to the OA and their caregivers. The primary care provider (PCP) should remember to be present and basically silent. This composure can occur at 5 levels:

- Hearing
- Understanding
- Retaining information
- Analyzing
- Active empathizing

Researchers at Ariadne studied 91 oncology clinicians and 278 patients at Dana-Farber Cancer Institute [23–25]. Findings helped create a communication quality improvement intervention (tool) for clinicians. The incorporation of advanced communication skills and techniques into the process of SICs is an important aspect with OAs and/or the ultimate EOL designated decision makers. SIC communication focuses on empathic skills related to prognostication and discussion about uncertainty related to serious illness and it incorporates the need to respond to OA/family/decision-maker emotions throughout the SICs [12,23,25,26].

As previously stated, an SIC requires a framework to guide the PCP. Intentionally and therapeutically listening to the OA story helps create a relational event with the APRN. Open-ended questions allow the OA and family members to tell their stories. A question to ask the OA is "what is in your bucket list?" or basically, "what would you love to have/do/see/experience before you leave this earth?" The bucket list is sometimes extraordinarily simplistic, such as an 88-year-old physician hospice patient who answered: (1) strawberry shake, (2) see my dogs, and (3) attend a (specific) college football game. All were arranged and enjoyed by the patient in his dying days. The third wish was to happen the day after he died peacefully and contentedly with a strawberry shake on his bedside table and 3 of his dogs on the bed with family members present. A beautiful ending to a well-lived life!

Ariadne Labs developed a guide to assist with the SIC flow (see Supplementary Data) [12,23,25].

The SIC involves key components to achieve a quality conversation and are presented in Box 2.

> **Box 2: Key components of a serious illness conversations**
> - Prepare for the conversation
> - Get notes, materials organized
> - Review and explore wishes, worries, fears, hopes, preferences of OAs and family/friends
> - Avoid distractions
> - Turn off pagers, cell phones, Ipad, computer
> - Mutual respect between all parties
> - Assessment/confirmation of understanding
> - Goal-directed conversation (not random)
> - Outcome and next steps are clear and agreed on
> - Active listening
> - Attentiveness
> - Response to emotion

CASE STUDY

History

NM is an 84-year-old African American woman who has resided in a skilled nursing facility for the last 5 years. The nursing staff have noticed increased forgetfulness and more episodes of shortness of breath in the previous 6 months. NM's current diagnoses are:

- COPD
- Dementia without behaviors
- HF
- Permanent pacemaker
- HTN
- Chronic kidney disease, stage 3
- Hyperlipidemia
- T2 diabetes mellitus (T2DM)
- Depression

NM had one emergency department (ED) visit for dyspnea on 04/12/19. The diagnosis was an exacerbation of HF. She is on the following medications:

- Daily, by mouth:
  - Lasix 20 mg
  - Zocor 20 mg
  - Metoprolol 50 mg
  - Remeron 15 mg
  - Cozaar 25 mg
- Daily, by inhalation device:
  - Spiriva 18 µg
- As necessary (prn):
  - Ipratropium bromide/Albuterol 0.5 mg/3 mL every 6 h prn for COPD

○ Norco 5/325 mg by mouth every 4 h prn for pain

NM is a widow; her daughter visits frequently. Her functional status has been declining. The Palliative Performance Scale (PPS) is a tool to measure the progression of a disease by the functional status of the OA. There are 5 functional domains:

- Ambulation—reduced, mainly sit/lie, mainly in bed, totally bed bound
- Activity and extent of disease—some, significant, extensive
- Self-care—requiring assistance (occasional, considerable, mainly) or total care
- Intake—normal, reduced, minimal
- Conscious level—full, drowsiness, coma

The 2019 PPS (version 2) can be found at https://consultgeri.org/try-this/general-assessment/issue-32.pdf.

NM's PPS score is 60% (see PPSv2) https://consultgeri.org/try-this/general-assessment/issue-32.pdf); she requires assistance with dressing, transfers, bathing, and eating—she sometimes refuses her evening meal. Her ambulation and appetite are reduced; cognition varies with some periods of increased confusion. The daughter became tearful during the discussion of possible surgery for the blockage in the left lower extremity (LLE). She would like all treatments to be given to her mother. She would like her mother to see a vascular surgeon for the coolness of the LLE. HF is progressing and NM requires oxygen 2 L/min through the nasal canal around the clock.

Assessment
A thorough review of systems and targeted physical assessment is required to determine NM's current medical status. Findings are represented in Box 3.

Diagnoses
1. Deep vein thrombosis left femoral artery
2. Acute chronic systolic HF

Differential diagnosis
Fracture left foot.

Diagnostic testing
1. Radiograph for left foot pain and coolness
2. oppler (same rationale as no. 1)
3. Complete blood count (CBC)

Diagnostic findings
1. Radiograph negative for a fracture
2. Doppler revealed thrombosis in left femoral artery
3. CBC nonremarkable, within normal limits for the resident

Treatment
1. Eliquis 10 mg by mouth twice a day for 7 days then convert to 5 mg by mouth daily
2. Morphine solution 20 mg per 5 mL, 0.25 mL every 4 hours for pain

Box 3: Review of systems and physical assessment findings

Pertinent review of systems:
- Shortness of breath
  - 3/10 scale
  - + shortness of breath during activities of daily living
  - Pain in LLE
  - 5/10 scale
  - Not well controlled with Norco
  - Denies headache, dizziness, lightheadedness, chest pain, nausea and vomiting, fever

Pertinent physical examination findings: no acute distress, lying in bed
- Vital signs:
  - Temp: 97.8°F
  - Pulse: 64 RRR
  - Resp: 16 eupneic
  - O_2 Sat: 90% on O_2 at 2 L/min via NC
  - BP: 132/82 left arm lying

Neck: negative JVD, bruits

CV: RRR S1 S2 S3; early systolic murmur at right apex

Lungs: diminished breath sounds, respiratory rate; negative for wheezes, rales, rhonchi

GI: nontender; soft bowel sounds × 4 quads; no organomegaly

Ext: +1 pedal edema bilateral ankles; left foot coolness and positive pain with palpation; bluish discoloration on left dorsalis pedis pulse, diminished, faint; no warmth or erythema bilateral legs

From the history, review of systems and assessment, the APRN is able to arrive at a diagnosis and develop a treatment plan.

Abbreviations: CP, chest pain; CV, cardiovascular; Ext, extremities; GI, gastrointenstinal; JVD, jugular vein distention; NC, nasal canal; RR, respiratory rate; RRR, regular rate and rhythm; S1, S2, and S3, first, and second, and third heart sound.

3. AD SICs with family
4. Vascular surgeon consultation

Management
1. SIC guide
2. American College of Cardiology (ACC)/American Heart Association (AHA) HF Classification (available at https://www.healio.com/cardiology/learn-the-heart/cardiology-review/topic-reviews/accaha-heart-failure-classification)
3. National Consensus Project (NCP) Clinical Practice Guidelines for Quality Palliative Care (4th ed.) (available at http://www.nationalcoalitionhpc.org/ncp/)

The conversation initiated with the daughter and the resident (the term to use with individuals living in LTC or other type of permanent home facility) to review the wishes on the treatment plan and AD. PC discussions include the entire family network—whoever is designated by the individual. The resident and daughter gave permission to review the clinical picture and address the ACP. The HCP (a gerontological nurse practitioner) reviewed the risk and benefits of having an amputation compared with comfort care. The HCP reviewed the following with NM's daughter and son:

- Goals of care
- Comfort care
- Functionality
- Longevity
- The difference between hospice and PC philosophies
- Trajectory of dementia, HF and T2DM
- NM's previously stated/written wishes, fears, preferences, and hope

The daughter and resident agreed to a do not resuscitate (DNR) order. NM's children went home to discuss the PC measures for NM.

The following day, the daughter again voiced she would like a vascular consult for her mother; NM stated she did not want an amputation. Everyone came to the agreement to respect their mother's wishes. A pain management plan was instituted and a consult with a vascular surgeon was scheduled to discuss the increased pain and thrombosis.

The final, mutually agreed on recommendation was to admit NM to the PC service and to transition to hospice at the EOL care. NM received oxygen for shortness of breath, morphine for pain management, and Ativan for restlessness. A depiction was shared with the daughter about the road to death (Fig. 2). Pictorials assist with the clarity of the comfort measure for family members who may feel they are abandoning their loved one.

NM was placed on hospice services on 06/01/19 and died peacefully on 09/10/19 with the guidance of the IDT approach. The skilled nursing home social worker contacted hospice to initiate services, as well as to support the family during the transcending of NM. Throughout the trajectory of serious illness, open-ended questions were used, and natural death occurred in the preferred setting of choice.

Byock reports "excellent care for people that are dying needs to be meticulous, methodical, proactive, and ongoing with regard to managing symptoms, conversation and planning" [11]. Caring for dying patients in the PCS and residents in LTC is a growing need as the aging population increases. Although dying at home may be the goal of most people, it is not always possible or affordable at this time. APRNs need to have an excellent understanding of chronic conditions and the dying process. Prognostication (foretelling future events based on EB knowledge) should be both ED and individualized. Evidence of quality of care in primary and LTC is an absolute necessity to provide true, transparent continuity of care.

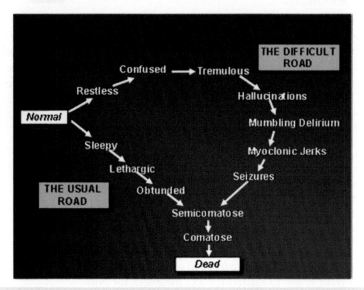

Fig. 2. Two roads to death. (*Adapted from* Freemon FR. Delirium and organic psychosis. In: Organic mental disease. Jamaica [NY]: SP Medical and Scientific Books; 1981. p. 81–94; with permission.)

BARRIERS OF EFFECTIVE COMMUNICATIONS

Acknowledgment of the numerous barriers that can prevent and interfere with effective communication needs to be addressed. First and foremost, all communication should be individually tailored to the OA and family level

---

Box 4: Key factors to prevent communication barriers

- Address issues related to patient/family goals of care and treatment preferences
- Analyze own communication (verbal and nonverbal) and possible interpretations of what the APRN says and does
  - Remember, body language and facial expression often speak louder than words to those in distress or at the EOL
- Respect cultural differences when discussing comfort, hospice, and palliative care
- Demonstrate knowledge of communication theory and principles within the context of hospice and palliative care
- Create an environment for effective communication
- Demonstrate therapeutic presence while maintaining professional boundaries
- Use appropriate principles and techniques to break bad news or engage in difficult conversations
- Elicit questions, concerns, or suggestions from the OA, family, faith leaders, IDT members, and so forth

Box 5: Self-reflection questions for the Advanced Practice Registered Nurse

- What do I believe about life and death?
- What are my preferences for EOL care if I am not able to participate in my own care?
- What are my feelings about a DNR order for individuals of any age?
  - Do I believe an OA with chronic comorbid incurable conditions should be a full code?
- What if someone I love asks me to be their designated decision-maker?
  - When the time comes, would I be able to carry out their wishes even though I disagree with them?
  - When could I or when could I not?
- Have I engaged in an SIC with my loved ones about myself? About them?
- Do I have an AD?
  - If YES—when was the last time you reviewed? (pick a special event—like birthday, anniversary, etc.—and review the AD every year on that special event day)
  - If NO—why?
- Do I clearly understand the concept of comfort care? Regulations, philosophy, framework, tools available, documentation, billing and reimbursement (for the patient and yourself)
  - Hospice care?
  - Palliative care?
- Am I able to explain to a patient and their family the philosophies of Hospice and Palliative care? Which comes first? Can they be done together? Can a patient start one or the other and then come off?
- Do I think patients should be informed of all aspects of their health? Or do I believe family can dictate level of knowledge and information that is to be shared? This would be for individuals over the age of 18
- Can you provide SICs based on the persons' need versus your own beliefs? In every situation?
- What if these questions were about the person you love most in the world—would your answers be different?
- Are you ready to have your own ACP conversation today? To talk to your loved ones about their AD?
  - If YES—terrific!
  - If NO—you need to consider how you can talk with patients and their families about life and death when you cannot face your own?
- Now—consider the rationale for your answers. Are you surprised?

of health literacy [21]. Mindfulness about OAs and their family ethnic and/or cultural beliefs can avoid leading to a misunderstanding of SICs. The presence of any impairment (visual or hearing loss, edentulous, aphasia, cognitive impairment) and psychological stress, such as depression or anxiety, along with spiritual distress, need to be evaluated and documented. Psychological concerns can be associated with psychiatric diagnoses and can alter OA and family's interactions and their ability to understand difficult news within an SIC. Box 4 presents information on how to prevent communication barriers.

IMPLICATIONS FOR PRACTICE

The APRN is in a pivotal role when working in a primary or LTC setting to guide and direct ACP and engage in SICs. The APRN needs to self-evaluate personal and professional feelings and knowledge of death and dying. Questions the APRN might ask of self are given in Box 5.

There are great materials and resources available to help you fill in your knowledge gaps—including from a spiritual or faith-based perspective. Understanding differences in culture/race/ethnicity and gender is also paramount in getting ready to have an SIC.

You can learn to do anything with comfort and grace. The first step is discovering yourself and your own beliefs. Then, explore options—talk to people who work with OAs and EOL on a regular basis. We can learn so much from our APRN colleagues and other health care professionals when we open our heart and minds to the mysteries of life and death. When the APRN is mindful and prepared, the impact one can make in the lives of patients and families at EOL is a gift—for you, from the individual. Sharing time at the end of days with those living the end of their journey can leave an indelible mark on your heart and spirit. You will have lived the art of nursing in a most remarkable manner. The APRN can help people to prepare their AD when healthy, talk about it over the years, and then help them to cross over from life to death in comfort and peace—in their way. This experience can be a celebration of a life lived and a death that was meaningful and full of life.

SUPPLEMENTARY DATA

Supplementary data related to this article can be found online at https://doi.org/10.1016/j.yfpn.2019.12.003.

References

[1] Centers for Disease Control and Prevention. Health communication basics. 2019. Available at: https://www.cdc.gov/healthcommunication/healthbasics/WhatIsHC.html. Accessed April 27, 2019.

[2] Browning D, Meyer E, Truog D, et al. Difficult conversations in health care: cultivating relational learning to address the hidden curriculum. Acad Med 2007;82(9):905–13.

[3] National Institutes of Health. World's older population grows dramatically. Available at: https://www.nih.gov/news-events/news-releases/worlds-older-population-grows-dramatically. Accessed April 27, 2019.

[4] Goodman D, Esty A, Fischer E, et al. Trend variations in end of life care for Medicare ben-eficiaries with severe chronic illness. 2011. Available at: http://dartmouthatlas.org/keyis-sues/issu.aspx?con=2944. Accessed April 27, 2019.

[5] Grossman S. Educating RNs regarding palliative care in long-term care generates positive outcomes for patients with end-stage chronic illness. J Hosp Palliat Nurs 2007;9(6):323–8.

[6] AgingStats.gov. Older Americans 2012: key indicators of well-being. 2012. Available at: http://www.agingstats.gov/agingstatsdotnet/Main_Site/Data/2012_Documents/Docs/EntireChartbook.pdf. Accessed September 10, 2019.

[7] Goodman DC, Fischer ES, Wennberg JE, et al. Tracking improvement in the care of chron-ically ill patients: a dartmouth atlas brief on Medicare beneficiaries near the end of life. 2013. Available at: www.dartmouthatlas.org4. Accessed September 10, 2019.

[8] Tulsky JA. Improving quality of care for serious illness: findings and recommendations of the Institute of Medicine report on dying in America. JAMA Intern Med 2015;175:840–1.

[9] Brazil K, Brink P, Kaasalainen S, et al. Knowledge and perceived competence among nurses caring for the dying in long-term care homes. Int J Palliat Nurs 2012;18(2):77–83.

[10] Sanders JJ, Curtis JR, Tulsky JA. Achieving goal-concordant care: a conceptual model and approach to measuring serious illness communication and its impact. J Palliat Med 2018;21(Suppl 2):S17–27.

[11] Moss AH, Lunney JR, Culp S, et al. Prognostic significance of the "surprise" question in can-cer patients. J Palliat Med 2010;13:837–40.

[12] Paladino J, Bernacki R, Neville BA. Evaluating an intervention to improve communication between oncology clinicians and patients with life-limiting cancer: a cluster-randomized clinical trial of the serious illness care program. JAMA Oncol 2019; https://doi.org/10.1001/jamaoncol.2019.0292.

[13] National Institute on Aging. Advance care planning: healthcare directives. Available at: https://www.nia.nih.gov/health/advance-care-planning-healthcare-directives. Accessed April 27, 2019.

[14] U.S. Government Site for Medicare. Advance care planning: is my test, item, or service covered?. Available at: https://www.medicare.gov/coverage/advance-care-planning. Accessed April 27, 2019.

[15] Lakin JR, Block SD, Billings JA, et al. Improving communication about serious illness in pri-mary care: a review. JAMA Intern Med 2016;176(9):1380–7.

[16] OM (Institute of Medicine). Dying in America: improving quality and honoring individual preferences near the end of life. Washington (DC): The National Academies Press; 2015. Available at: https://www.nap.edu/catalog/18748/dying-in-america-improving-quality-and-honoring-individual-preferences-near. Accessed June 22, 2019.

[17] World Health Organization. WHO definition of palliative care. Available at: https://www.who.int/cancer/palliative/definition/en/. Accessed April 27, 2019.

[18] World Health Organization (WHO). 2012 definition of palliative care. Available at: http://www.who.int/cancer/palliative/definition/enl. Accessed April 27, 2019.

[19] American Nurses Association. Nursing: scope and standards of practice. 3rd edition. Silver Spring (MD): Nursebooks.org; 2015.

[20] American Nurses Association, Hospice and Palliative Nurses Association. Palliative nursing: scope and standards of practice—an essential resource for hospice and palliative nurses. 5th edition. Silver Spring (MD): American Nurses Association and Hospice and Palli-ative Nurses Association; 2014.

[21] National Consensus Project for Quality Palliative Care. Clinical practice guidelines for qual-ity palliative care. 4th edition. Richmond (VA): National Coalition for Hospice and Palliative Care; 2018. Available at: https://www.nationalcoalitionhpc.org.

[22] Emanuel LL, von Gunten CF, Ferris FD, editors. The EPEC curriculum: education for physi-cians on end-of-life care. The EPEC project. 1999. Available at: http://www.epeconline.-net/EPEC/Webpages/ph.cfm 1999. Accessed August, 2019.

[23] Ariadne Labs. Serious illness care program, communication in serious illness: an innovative approach to clinical care and quality improvement. Boston: Ariadne Labs; 2016.

[24] Byock I. The best care possible, a physician's quest to transform care through the end of life. New York: Penguin Group; 2012. p. 125–64.

[25] Kelley AS, Morrison RS. Palliative care for the seriously ill. N Engl J Med 2015;373(8):747–55.

[26] Bernacki RE, Block SD. Communication about serious illness care goals: a review and synthesis of best practices. JAMA Intern Med 2014;174:1994–2003.

Advances in Family Practice Nursing 2 (2020) 37–47

ADVANCES IN FAMILY PRACTICE NURSING

The Role of the Primary Care Provider in Work-up and Management of Parkinson Disease

Abby Luck Parish, DNP, AGPCNP-BC, GNP-BC, FNAP*,
Jennifer Kim, DNP, GNP-BC, GS-C, FNAP, FAANP

Vanderbilt School of Nursing, 461 21st Avenue South, Nashville, TN 37240, USA

Keywords
• Parkinson disease • Primary care • Nurse practitioner

Key points

• The older adult population is rapidly growing, and the incidence of diseases associated with advanced age is increasing accordingly.

• Parkinson disease is a progressive neurodegenerative disease affecting approximately 6.3 million individuals globally in 2015.

• Emerging evidence suggests that dopamine depletion in Parkinson disease is a secondary effect of the development of α-synuclein–containing Lewy bodies, suggesting future opportunities for biomarkers and/or therapies.

• Primary care nurse practitioners should be prepared to identify and assess presenting and/or cardinal features of Parkinson disease, including tremor, bradykinesia, rigidity, and postural instability.

• Primary care nurse practitioners play an integral role in the management of associated symptoms of Parkinson disease, such as constipation, depression, and pain, throughout the disease trajectory.

INTRODUCTION

Although Parkinson disease (PD) was first described by James Parkinson more than 200 years ago, recent changes in population demographics, understanding of disease pathology, and diagnostic criteria necessitate that primary care nurse practitioners (NPs) revisit and renew their understanding of and approach to patients with PD. PD is a progressive neurodegenerative disease whose incidence and prevalence has been increasing globally. Advanced age is the

*Corresponding author. E-mail address: Abby.parish@vanderbilt.edu

https://doi.org/10.1016/j.yfpn.2019.12.004
2589-420X/20/

main risk factor for PD, with disease incidence increasing sharply at the age of 60 years, and peaking between age 70 and 79 years [1,2]. It is the second most common neurodegenerative disease in the older adult population and the fastest growing of all neurologic disorders internationally [3,4]. In 2015, approximately 6.3 million people across the world had a diagnosis of PD [2,3]. This number is expected to increase to 12.9 million by the year 2040, with increased prevalence in the western Pacific region accounting for the biggest change [3,5]. The increasing incidence and prevalence of PD is likely caused by increased quality of health care and the expanding older adult population [3].

Motor and nonmotor symptoms of disease become more pronounced as PD progresses, ultimately resulting in significant physical and functional disability. Direct costs of PD are high, with an estimated $14 billion incurred in 2010 [6]. Indirect costs, including decreased overall productivity, reduced workforce contributions, overall difficulty in achieving job functions, and work absenteeism, were likely responsible for the loss of an additional $6.3 billion [6]. Approximately 15% of individuals with PD live in long-term care facilities, because of increased demands for assistance with physical care [6].

PATHOPHYSIOLOGY

The exact cause of PD is not known. Approximately 90% of PD diagnoses are idiopathic, whereas 10% of all newly diagnosed cases are thought to have been inherited [7]. The precise pathogenesis of idiopathic PD is unknown, but it is hypothesized to be caused by a combination of genetic vulnerability, aging, and environmental factors [1,3]. More than 40 risk loci for PD have been identified in genome-wide association studies [8]. Causative mutations associated with PD (*LRRK2, SNCA, VPS35, Parkin, PINK1, DJ1,* and *GBA*) are much rarer than risk loci, accounting for only 5% to 10% of all PD cases [9]. The pathologic features of familial PD, age of onset, and severity of symptoms are heterogeneous and depend on the specific genetic mutation, with some mutations yielding a more pronounced and aggressive form of disease [10]. Although current literature examining the relationship between specific mutations with response to PD treatment is scarce, genetic profiling may be relevant in the future, as clinicians aim to provide personalized care and treatment.

Clinicians commonly associate PD with dopamine depletion, because that is the physiologic basis for many of the observable symptoms of illness. However, there is a growing body of research to support the notion that dopamine depletion is a secondary result of disease and the primary pathophysiologic change in PD is the development of α-synuclein–containing Lewy bodies [11]. α-Synuclein is a protein that is normally occurring; in individuals with PD, there is an excess of α-synuclein, resulting in the development of α-synuclein–containing Lewy bodies [11]. Lewy bodies form first in the anterior olfactory nucleus and brainstem, and then progress upward through the brain [11,12]. When α-synuclein–containing Lewy bodies progress to the substantia nigra, dopamine depletion occurs and the person becomes symptomatic [11,12].

Thus, there is a prodromal phase of illness during which significant pathophysiologic changes are occurring, although patients experience minimal symptoms. Hawkes and colleagues [12] proposed a timeline based on this understanding of pathophysiology, which has been adopted as the understood model of disease progression. The model includes an average 20-year prodromal period followed by a symptomatic period [12]. The symptomatic period is most commonly staged using the criteria published by Hoehn and Yahr [13] in 1967, which include 5 stages of disease, representing progression from mild to severe symptoms.

HISTORY

During the prodromal phase of illness, the most commonly experienced symptoms include hyposmia, constipation, bladder dysfunction, depression, and/or obesity [12]. The subsequent emergence of motor symptoms, including bradykinesia, rest tremor, and/or rigidity, typically prompts individuals to seek medical care. The patient's history of unilateral emergence and presentation of motor symptoms is a distinguishing feature of the disease. As PD progresses, both sides of the body are affected, but the side on which symptoms begin is typically affected to a greater extent than the contralateral side [14].

Although motor symptoms typically prompt patients to seek care, and are also responsible for disease-related disability, nonmotor symptoms are also prominent throughout the disease course [12,14]. Cardinal features of PD include tremor, bradykinesia, rigidity, and postural instability. There are additional features commonly found in the disease, but their presence is variable among patients with PD.

ASSESSMENT

PD is a clinical diagnosis. A thorough history and physical examination (PE) is essential. Clinicians should ensure that correct assessment techniques are used to confirm or rule out a diagnosis of PD when a patient presents with its clinical features (Table 1).

Published in 2008, the Movement Disorder Society Unified Parkinson's Disease Rating Scale (MDS-UPDRS) is a revised version of the original UPDRS that was developed in the 1980s [15]. It is the most widely used rating scale to assess the severity and progression of motor and nonmotor symptoms and includes clinician evaluation as well as patient and caregiver input within the following domains:

- Motor and nonmotor experiences of daily living
- Motor examination
- Motor complications

Although the time for patient-reported outcomes may vary, it is estimated to take less than 30 minutes to administer [15]. The MDS-UPRDS is available for free download at www.movementdisorders.org.

Table 1
Physical assessment

Clinical feature	Assessment techniques	Examination findings Supporting diagnosis
Tremor	• Ensure limb is at rest and fully relaxed • May observe throughout examination and/or with use distraction	• 4-Hz to 6-Hz tremor in a fully resting limb • Tremor is suppressed during initiation of movement

Bradykinesia	• Ask patient to complete following repeated movements:
	  ○ Finger tapping
	  ○ Hand movements
	  ○ Pronation/supination movements
	  ○ Toe tapping
	  ○ Foot tapping
		• Slowness of movement and reduced amplitude or speed as movements are continued
		• Limb bradykinesia must be documented for diagnosis of PD

Rigidity	• Slow passive range of motion • Patient must be in relaxed position • Clinician should manipulate limbs and neck	Leadpipe resistance (resistance to passive movement not related to velocity; or the inability to relax)

Data from Postuma, RB, Berg, D, Stern, M, et al. MDS clinical diagnostic criteria for Parkinson's disease. Mov Disord. 2015;30(12):1591 – 1599.

DIAGNOSTIC TESTING

Primary care NPs may consider laboratory work and/or imaging if it would contribute to ruling out another diagnosis, but, at this time, the diagnosis of PD is made from history and PE findings; no confirmatory biomarkers or imaging are advised. Researchers have sought to identify biomarkers for diagnostic confirmation because early detection of illness during the prodromal phase could be useful for neuroprotective trials and/or treatment [16]. Based on the emerging conceptualization of PD as a synucleinopathy, α-synuclein species and aggregates in the blood and cerebrospinal fluid respectively are currently under consideration [16]. At this time, there is neither an easily accessible nor broadly recommended set of biomarkers for patients with suspected disease, but clinicians should continue to monitor the evidence for emerging options.

DIAGNOSIS

Although the MDS-UPDRS investigators acknowledge the prevalence and burden of nonmotor symptoms of PD, diagnosis continues to be from motor symptoms [17]. Specifically, to be diagnosed with general parkinsonism, a person must have bradykinesia plus at least 1 of the other 2 cardinal symptoms, rigidity or rest tremor [17]. The criteria then provide guidance to distinguish between PD and other causes of parkinsonism, including red flags that suggest other causes of parkinsonism and supportive criteria that contribute to a PD diagnosis [17]. The most supportive criteria for a PD diagnosis is a clear and dramatic benefit from a trial of dopaminergic therapy (ie, levodopa/carbidopa) [17]. A trial of levodopa/carbidopa is often undertaken during the diagnostic process and, if the person has a positive and sustained response, this may confirm the PD diagnosis.

During the work-up and diagnostic phase, the primary care NP is advised to complete a thorough examination, and, if concern for PD or a related condition exists, the NP should consider a referral to neurology for comprehensive history, PE, and diagnostic communication. Patients with PD receiving care with a neurologist may experience improvement of some clinical outcomes, including time to skilled nursing placement, risk of hip fracture and even mortality [18], and an equivocal number of overall hospitalizations [19]. Health disparities in accessing neurology care exist, with women and people of color being less likely to receive care [18].

DIFFERENTIAL DIAGNOSIS

Essential tremor is a benign condition that is commonly seen by primary clinicians and may be mistaken for a resting tremor of PD. Compared with the resting tremor of PD, in which tremor typically begins unilaterally and worsens at rest, essential tremor is more commonly bilateral and worsens during fine motor activity [20]. There are multiple causes of parkinsonism that may mimic PD, most of which are more common with advanced age (Table 2). It is important to rule out these causes, because they require alternate treatment plans, often with referral to a specialist.

TREATMENT OF MOTOR SYMPTOMS

At this time, there are no curative or neuroprotective treatment options for PD. Clinicians may anticipate that recent advances in understanding of pathophysiologic changes of disease could ultimately translate into development of neuroprotective therapies, which could ideally be applied during the dormant phase of illness. Until that time, the treatment of PD is symptomatic. It is important for clinicians to be aware that the motor symptoms of PD are experienced as being very bothersome or uncomfortable for patients [21]. In addition, motor symptoms are ultimately responsible for significant functional impairment and disability. Thus, optimal pharmacologic management of motor symptoms is essential for patient quality of life (QOL) and functionality. Pharmacologic management of motor symptoms is often driven or directed by a neurologist. By understanding principles of management, primary care NPs can play a role in monitoring symptom relief, titrating medications, and referring back to neurology for advanced adjustments as needed. Symptomatic therapy for motor symptoms of PD is intended to promote available dopamine in the substantia nigra (Table 3).

Initial pharmacotherapy with levodopa/carbidopa is typically associated with significant relief of motor symptoms. However, over time, the magnitude and duration of symptom relief associated with levodopa/carbidopa declines [22,26]. A common initial management strategy is dose titrations and schedule adjustments to optimize symptom-free time [23]. After several years of

Table 2
Secondary and atypical Parkinsonism

Type of parkinsonism	Causes	History and PE findings
Secondary parkinsonism	Toxins	• Exposure to carbon monoxide, cyanide, manganese, organic solvents, or other toxins
	Medications • Dopamine receptor blockers • Dopamine storage depletors	• Recent exposure to typical and atypical antipsychotics, metoclopramide, reserpine
	Structural lesions in brain • Hydrocephalus • Chronic subdural hematoma • Tumor	• Focal neurologic signs • New onset of clinical triad: urinary incontinence, gait instability, and cognitive loss
	Head trauma • Isolated or repeated	• Visible signs of trauma • History of fall with head strike • History of contact sport
Atypical parkinsonism	Progressive supranuclear palsy	• Loss of ocular movements • Myoclonus • Falling or freezing of gait (in early disease)
	Multiple system atrophy	• Cerebellar ataxia • Pronounced postural hypotension or autonomic dysfunction, unrelated to medication • Excessive drooling • Dystonia induced with low dose levodopa
	Corticobasal syndrome	• Pronounced unilateral rigidity • Myoclonus

Data from Halter, JB, Ouslander, JG, Studenski, S, et al. Hazzards's Geriatric Medicine and Gerontology, 7th ed. New York, New York: McGraw Hill; 2017; and Ahlskog, JE. Diagnosis and differential diagnosis of Parkinson's disease and parkinsonism. Parkinsonism & Related Disorders. 2000;7(1):63-70.

levodopa/carbidopa therapy, patients may begin to experience 2 common medication effects: off-time and dyskinesias [22,26]. The time to these effects may vary and is thought to be dose related, so it is advised that, throughout the course of illness, patients take the lowest tolerable dose in order to maximize time before off-time and dyskinesias emerge [22,23]. Off-time captures the notion that, in later disease, patients experience periods of bothersome motor symptoms between doses of levodopa/carbidopa that do not respond to adjustments in dose or dosing frequency [22]. Dyskinesias are involuntary, choreiform-type movements that may affect the limbs, head, and trunk, and they may be reduced by reducing the levodopa/carbidopa dose [22]. The occurrence of bothersome off-time and/or dyskinesias is an appropriate juncture to refer patients back to the neurology setting for troubleshooting.

Table 3 Pharmacologic treatment of motor symptoms in Parkinson disease [22–25]		
Symptom	Treatment options	Comments on use
Tremor, bradykinesia, rigidity	Dopamine	Mainstay of PD treatment
	Extended release	Reduces/improves motor fluctuations and troublesome dyskinesias
	Immediate release	Long-term treatment associated with motor fluctuations and dyskinesias
	Duopa	Intestinal gel; for use in patients with enteral feeding
	Dopamine agonist	May be used as first line or in conjunction with levodopa
	Ropinirole and pramipexole	Extended-release and immediate-release preparations
	Rotigotine	Transdermal preparation
	Apomorphine	SQ preparation; used for maintenance therapy or for off-time rescue
Persistent tremor (with use of dopamine or dopamine-agonist treatment)	+ Clozapine	Effectiveness lacks of strong evidence. Risk for serious side effects (agranulocytosis)
	Consider DBS	Typically reserved for later stages of PD
Freezing of gait	Methylphenidate	Off-label use
	Atomoxetine	Off-label use
Bradykinesia, motor fluctuations, increased off-time (with use of dopamine)	↑ Dopamine dose	
	+ Dopamine agonist	
	+ COMT inhibitor (tolcapone, entacapone)	Tolcapone: monitor LFTs Entacapone: monitor for nausea and orthostasis
	+ MAO B inhibitor (rasagiline, safinamide, selegiline)	Many drug interactions
	Consider DBS for refractory fluctuations	Typically reserved for later stages of PD
Postural instability or gait impairment, despite dopamine treatment	Amantadine	May be used in early and late PD Monitor for CNS side effects Taper off when stopping
	CI	Rivastigmine is CI of choice
Dyskinesia	Amantadine	—
	↓ Dopamine dose	—
	Consider clozapine	—

Abbreviations: CI, cholinesterase inhibitor; CNS, central nervous system; COMT, catechol-O-methyltransferase; DBS, deep brain stimulation; LFTs, liver function tests; MAO, monoamine oxidase; SQ, subcutaneous.

Deep brain stimulation is a device-assisted treatment option that is usually reserved for those who have significant motor symptoms and drug-related dyskinesias and those in the later stages of PD [23]. Deep brain stimulation is surgical stimulation of the subthalamic nucleus or globus pallidus internus, which results in relief of motor symptoms, less off-time, and fewer dyskinesias [22]. This invasive procedure may result in adverse effects, including infection, bleeding, stroke, apathy, and suicidality, so its role is limited to later disease in patients for whom levodopa is less effective [22].

MANAGEMENT

Primary care NPs often collaborate with neurologists in the care of patients with PD. In certain situations, or in areas with limited access to health care, primary care NPs may be the sole providers for patients with PD. More than 40% of older adults with PD who live in wealthy countries do not see a neurologist [3]. When collaborating care with a neurologist, primary care NPs are responsible for monitoring, assessing, and managing common PD-associated symptoms (Table 4).

Primary care NPs must recognize and recommend community resources for patients with PD. NPs can provide patients and family members with information about local resources such as group-based therapy, physical activity centers, and centers for older adults. Patients and families may also appreciate referrals to online entities such as the American Parkinson Disease Association (https://www.apdaparkinson.org/) or the Parkinson's Foundation (https://www.parkinson.org/), which contain education and resources for disease management.

HEALTH PROMOTION

Patients with PD should be encouraged to be physical active [23]. Physical activity may reduce falls in persons with PD, particularly if the program focuses on balance and/or strength training and involves greater than 3 h/wk [27,28]. Physical activity may be associated with outcomes such as increased QOL, improved mood, and pain relief [29,30]. Physical activity may promote socialization and yield improvements in self-efficacy. Many patients with PD have other chronic health conditions, for which physical activity is beneficial. NPs should encourage physical activity in patients with early and moderate PD, being mindful that a referral to physical and occupational therapy may be warranted for a prescribed physical activity plan that takes the patient's functional limitations into account [23].

A balanced, high-fiber diet and adequate hydration should be encouraged because patients with PD commonly have constipation related to the disease process and to medications used to treat the disease [23]. Because of the pharmacokinetics of levodopa, patients should be encouraged to separate levodopa from protein, with consideration to consolidation of protein at the final meal of the day [23]. Modifications to food texture are often made in the later stages of disease because of problems with dysphagia.

Patients' many needs related to PD often eclipse other important preventive care measures. Preventive care and screenings should be encouraged. Similar to care for all older adults, NPs must consider each patient's goals of care when making recommendations [23].

Table 4
Associated symptoms of Parkinson disease

Associated symptom	Assessment/management strategies	At-risk geriatric syndromes
Orthostatic hypotension	• Abdominal binders • TED hose • Medications: consider fludrocortisone, midodrine, pyridostigmine	Falls
Constipation	• ↑ Fiber • ↑ Hydration • Daily Miralax	Delirium
Dementia	• Consider trial of cholinesterase inhibitor (rivastigmine) • Supportive care	• Falls • Malnutrition • Sleep disturbances • Polypharmacy • Frailty • Polypharmacy
Depression	• Cognitive behavior therapy • SSRI or SNRI • Consider trial of pramipexole • Tailor to the individual	• Malnutrition • Failure to thrive • Sleep disorders
Dysphagia	Increase risk of infection	• Malnutrition • Weight loss
Pain	• Exercise • Physical therapy	• Falls • Malnutrition
Psychosis/ hallucinations	• Careful reduction of antiparkinsonian drugs, anticholinergic medications, anxiolytics, amantadine • Reduce polypharmacy • Consider pimavanserin • Consider quetiapine or clozapine (requires monitoring) if needed • Avoid all other antipyschotics	• Falls • Delirium • Polypharmacy
Sleep disorders	• Consider melatonin or clonazepam (only in those with dementia) • Use low doses of sedating antidepressants (eg, trazodone)	• Falls • Delirium

Abbreviations: SNRI, serotonin norepinephrine reuptake inhibitor; SSRI, selective serotonin reuptake inhibitor; TED, thromboembolic deterrent.

Data from Grimes, D, Fitzpatrick, M, Gordon, J, et al. Canadian guideline for Parkinson disease. CMAJ. 2019;191:E989-1004 and Reuben, DB, Herr, KA, Pacala, JT, et al. Geriatrics at Your Fingertips, 21st ed. New York, NY; The American Geriatrics Society, 2019.

SUMMARY

Primary care NPs play an important role in the management of PD by assessing presenting symptoms, referring patients to neurology for diagnosis and comanagement of motor symptoms, monitoring symptoms, and providing education and treatment of PD's associated symptoms. It is critical that NPs are aware of the emerging understanding of PD as a synucleinopathy that has a lengthy prodromal period with motor symptoms appearing at the time that α-synuclein–containing Lewy bodies and resultant dopamine depletion progress to the substantia nigra. Primary care NPs can play a key role in the identification and assessment of early PD symptoms. Although treatment of motor symptoms may be largely managed in the neurology setting, primary care NPs can provide supportive care for associated symptoms throughout the PD trajectory. By providing supportive and holistic care, NPs may optimize the functionality and wellbeing of persons with PD.

Disclosure
The authors have nothing to disclose.

References
[1] Pang SY, Ho PW, Liu HF, et al. The interplay of aging, genetics and environmental factors in the pathogenesis of Parkinson's disease. Transl Neurodegener 2019;8(23): 1–11.

[2] Pringsheim T, Jette NT, Frolkis A, et al. The prevalence of Parkinson's disease: A systematic review and meta-analysis. Mov Disord 2014;29:1583–90.

[3] Dorsey ER, Bloem BR. The Parkinson pandemic – a call to action. JAMA Neurol 2018;75(1): 9–10.

[4] Halter JB, Ouslander JG, Studenski S, et al. Hazzards's geriatric medicine and gerontology. 7th edition. New York: McGraw Hill; 2017.

[5] Lim SY, Tan AH, Ahmad-Annuar A, et al. Parkinson's disease in the Western Pacific Region. Lancet Neurol 2019;18(9):865–8796.

[6] Kowal SL1, Dall TM, Chakrabarti R, et al. The current and projected economic burden of Parkinson's disease in the United States. Mov Disord 2013;28(3):311–8.

[7] Dexter DT, Jenner P. Parkinson disease: from pathology to molecular disease mechanisms. Free Radic Biol Med 2013;62:132–44.

[8] Chang D, Nalls MA, Hallgrimsdottir IB. A meta-analysis of genome-wide association studies identifies 17 new Parkinson's disease risk loci. Nat Genet 2017;49(10): 1511–6.

[9] Kim CY, Alcalay R. Genetic forms of Parkinson's disease. Semin Neurol 2017;37:135–46.

[10] Bonifati V. Genetics of Parkinson's disease- state of the art, 2013. Parkinsonism Relat Disord 2014;20(S1):S23–8.

[11] Fahn S. The 200-year journey of Parkinson disease: reflecting on the past and looking towards the future. Parkinsonism Relat Disord 2018;46(1):S1–5.

[12] Hawkes CH, Del Tredici K, Braak H. A timeline for Parkinson's disease. Parkinsonism Relat Disord 2010;16:79–84.

[13] Hoehn MM, Yahr MD. Parkinsonism: onset, progression, and mortality. Neurology 1967;17(5):427–42.

[14] Poewe W. The natural history of Parkinson's disease. J Neurol 2006;253:VII/2–6.

[15] Goetz CG, Tilley BC, Shaftman SR, et al. Movement Disorder Society-sponsored revision of the Unified Parkinson's Disease Rating Scale (MDS-PPDRS): Scale presentation and clinimetric testing results. Mov Disord 2008;23(15):2129–70.

[16] Parnetti L, Gaetani L, Eusebi P, et al. CSF and blood biomarkers for Parkinson's disease. Lancet Neurol 2019;18:573–86.

[17] Postuma RB, Berg D, Stern M, et al. MDS clinical diagnostic criteria for Parkinson's disease. Mov Disord 2015;30(12):1591–9.

[18] Willis AW, Schootman M, Evanoff BA, et al. Neurologist care in Parkinson's disease: A utilization, outcomes and survival study. Neurology 2011;77:851–7.

[19] Willis AW, Schootman M, Tran R, et al. Neurologist-associated reduction in PD-related hospitalizations and health care expenditures. Neurology 2012;79:1774–80.

[20] Haubenberger D, Hallett M. Essential tremor. N Engl J Med 2018;378(19):1802–10.

[21] Uebelacker LA, Epstein-Lubow G, Lewis T, et al. A survey of Parkinson's disease patients: most bothersome symptoms and coping preferences. J Parkinsons Dis 2014;4(4):717–23.
[22] Cabreira V, Soares-da-Silva P, Massano J. Contemporary options for the management of motor complications in Parkinson's Disease: Updated clinical review. Drugs 2019;79: 593–608.
[23] Grimes D, Fitzpatrick M, Gordon J, et al. Canadian guideline for Parkinson disease. CMAJ 2019;191:E989–1004.
[24] Reuben DB, Herr KA, Pacala JT, et al. Geriatrics at Your Fingertips. 21st edition. New York: The American Geriatrics Society; 2019.
[25] Tarakad A, Jancovic J. Diagnosis and management of Parkinson's disease. Semin Neurol 2017;37:118–26.
[26] LeWitt PA, Fahn S. Levodopa therapy for Parkinson disease: A look backward and forward. Neurology 2016;86(14 Supplement 1):S3–12.
[27] Shen X, Wong-Yu IS, Mak MK. Effects of exercise on falls, balance, and gait ability in Parkinson's Disease: A meta-analysis. Neurohabil Neural Repair 2016;30(6):512–27.
[28] Sherrington C, Michaleff ZA, Fairhall N, et al. Exercise to prevent falls in older adults: an updated systematic review and meta-analysis. Br J Sports Med 2017;51:1750–8.
[29] Canning CG, Sherrington C, Lord SR, et al. Exercise for falls prevention in Parkinson disease. Neurology 2015;84(3):304–12.
[30] Mak MK, Wong-Yu IS, Shen X, et al. Long-term effects of exercise and physical therapy in people with Parkinson disease. Nat Rev Neurol 2017;13:689–703.

Advances in Family Practice Nursing 2 (2020) 49–62

ADVANCES IN FAMILY PRACTICE NURSING

ELSEVIER
MOSBY

Irregularly Irregular
Atrial Fibrillation in Primary Care

Mary Jane Cook, PhD, RN, FNP-BC

Michigan State University College of Nursing, 1355 Bogue Street, Life Sciences Building, Room A110, East Lansing, MI 48824, USA

Keywords
- Atrial fibrillation • Older adults • Primary care

Key points
- The incidence of AF is highest in older adults. AF results from changes due to normal aging combined with co-morbid chronic conditions.
- Thromboembolism and reduced cardiac output are the leading causes of morbidity and mortality.
- Thromboembolism prevention is guided by patient risk factors for stroke and hemorrhage. Risk is determined using the CHA2DS2-VASc and HAS-BLED scoring systems.
- Rate control is the priority in AF management. Rhythm control is considered based on patient preference, co-morbidities, and hemodynamics.
- The primary care NP plays an important role in identifying AF, ordering appropriate testing, and shared decision-making to optimize health and quality of life.

A trial fibrillation (AF) is the most common cardiac arrhythmia in older adults. In 2017 there were between 2.7 and 6.1 million people diagnosed with AF in the United States [1]. The prevalence of older adults with AF is increasing and the number is expected to double by 2050 [2]. The morbidity and mortality from AF caused by heart failure (HF) and ischemic stroke results in approximately 750,000 hospitalizations and 130,000 deaths per year. Between 1990 and 2010, there was a 2-fold mortality increase from AF [3]. AF costs the United States health care system nearly 6 billion dollars per year [1].

The incidence of AF increases with age, placing the burden of the disease on older adults. In fact, risk of AF doubles in each decade of life. Primary care

E-mail address: cookma@msu.edu

https://doi.org/10.1016/j.yfpn.2020.01.009

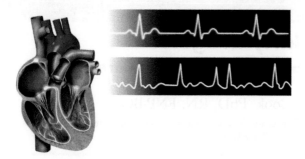

Fig. 1. Sinus rhythm in comparison with atrial fibrillation. (*From* Wikimedia Commons. Available: https://commons.wikimedia.org/wiki/Category:Atrial_fibrillation#/media/File:Atrial_Fibrillation.jpg. Accessed October 10, 2019.)

physicians (PCPs) can have 10% of their patient population aged 80 to 84 years with the disease [4]. In older adults with chronic comorbid conditions, AF contributes to deterioration in cognition, function, increased falls, disengagement, and inappropriate polypharmacy [4,5]. In addition, fatigue, anxiety about the condition, and lack of sleep all contribute to a reduction in age-related quality of life (QoL) [6].

PATHOPHYSIOLOGY

Risk factors play a fundamental and important role in the pathophysiology of AF [3]. AF is a supraventricular arrhythmia with uncoordinated electrical activity of the atria. The atrial impulses fire 400 to 600 times per minute [7]. The chaotic electrical impulses from multiple foci result in an irregularly irregular ventricular rhythm, leading to atrial impulses conducted unpredictably to the ventricle. The transmission of the fibrillatory waves intermittently to the ventricles is blocked by the atrial-ventricular node (Fig. 1). The electrocardiographic characteristics of AF include (Fig. 2):

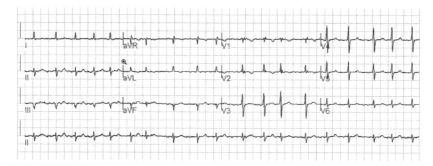

Fig. 2. Atrial fibrillation demonstrated on 12-lead ECG. Note the irregular rhythm and baseline of the fibrillatory waves.

1. Lack of a visible atrial impulse or p wave
2. A wavy undulating pattern called fibrillatory waves at baseline
3. Irregular spacing of the ventricular impulses

AF is classified according to the duration of episodes as paroxysmal, persistent, long-standing persistent, and permanent [8,9]. Clinical outcomes from evidence-based (EB) and targeted therapies relate to duration of the AF. Paroxysmal atrial fibrillation (PAF), also referred to as recurrent or intermittent AF, is defined by 2 episodes that terminate spontaneously within 7 days, and can recur at any time [10]. Persistent AF generally lasts for more than 7 days. Long-standing persistent AF has been sustained for more than 12 months. Both paroxysmal and persistent AF can occur concomitantly. Permanent AF is a clinical designation rather than one based on duration of the episodes. The classification is based on the shared decision of the patient and PCP to discontinue efforts to convert the arrhythmia to normal sinus rhythm (NSR).

Causes

The causes of AF are attributable to several mechanisms within the cardiovascular system. For most individuals, AF is a combination of aging, acquired disease, and genetic risk factors; it is often difficult to pinpoint the exact cause. Advancing age is the primary risk factor for AF. Older adults lose cardiac muscle cells as they age normally and fibrotic tissue forms as a result [11]. In addition, older adults are more likely to have coexisting acquired diseases such as hypertension, diabetes, or atherosclerosis. These coexisting diseases contribute to the fibrosis, inflammation, and remodeling of the cardiac muscle. The fibrotic tissue inhibits the ability of the electrical impulses to propagate, normally leading to AF.

The autonomic nervous system plays a major role in triggering and sustaining AF. The atria are innervated by both sympathetic and parasympathetic axons. The electrical properties of the atrial impulses, such as rate and refractory period, are changed by autonomic nerve function. Vagal stimulation can prevent AF, whereas the sympathetic stimulation of high-intensity endurance training can provoke it [11]. The incidence of AF also increases in sleep apnea, a result of sympathetic nervous system (SNS) activation.

Intracellular calcium and ion-channel dysfunction are also factors in the risk of AF. Abnormal calcium handling by the cardiac muscle leads to an increase in spontaneous electrical activity. Ion-channel dysfunction changes the electrical characteristics of the atrial impulses leading to a prolonged action potential, enhancing the ectopic activity. Metabolic changes, cardiac muscle stressors, and catecholamine levels affect both intracellular calcium and ion-channel regulation [7].

Genetic factors play a role in AF. The likelihood of AF increases by 40% if a family member has, or has had, the arrhythmia [8]. This hereditary AF link most often occurs before the age of 66 years [12]. Common genetic variants that predispose individuals to AF are found in approximately one-third of all AF patients [13]. Numerous genetic variants, with a variety of mechanisms of action, are linked to AF. Since genetic testing has limited value in risk assessment, it is currently not recommended as part of EB clinical care.

Hemodynamics
AF causes a reduction in cardiac output. Hemodynamic consequences are the result of:

1. Uncontrolled ventricular rate
2. Loss of effective atrial contraction
3. Variable filling time of the ventricles
4. Activation of the SNS

The rapid chaotic atrial impulses are conducted to the ventricles, increasing heart rate. The ventricles have less time to fill with blood and cardiac output is reduced. Loss of effective atrial contraction reduces the blood volume in the ventricle at the end of diastole. Atrial contraction contributes 20% to 30% of ventricular end-diastolic volume [8]. The irregular ventricular rate in AF changes the duration of ventricular diastole. Ventricular filling time is unpredictable and reduced, especially with higher heart rates. Finally, activation of the SNS in AF increases the strength of ventricular contraction and increases the ventricular rate.

DIAGNOSIS
PCPs are often the first to discover AF during cardiac auscultation. The clinician should have a high index of suspicion on hearing an irregularly irregular rhythm. A suspicion of AF diagnosis, based on cardiac assessment and pulse rate, should always be confirmed with a single 12-lead electrocardiogram (ECG). An ECG confirms the diagnosis of AF. According to Gutierrez and Blanchard [14], a normal ECG does not necessarily rule out the presence of AF; a PAF rhythm may not be captured. When the PCP believes AF is present, a Holter monitor (24-h recording) or event monitor (7- to 30-day recording) may be necessary. The prognosis for AF is primarily determined by stroke risk [15].

Symptomatology
Patients with AF can be symptomatic or asymptomatic. Older adults are often asymptomatic, or if they report vague symptoms PCPs attribute symptoms to normal aging. Symptoms are often related to either a rapid heart rate or decreased cardiac output. Heart rate–related symptoms include:

- Palpitations
- Lightheadedness or dizziness
- Near syncope

Chest pain, dyspnea, exercise intolerance, orthopnea, edema, and fatigue are related to reduction in cardiac output. Patients who are symptomatic with tachycardia and hypotension should receive hospital emergency care. It is unsafe for older adults with near syncope to be sent home from the primary care office.

History

A comprehensive assessment of the older adult is essential. The history should focus on cardiac risk factors, family history, comorbidities, function, social status, and possible triggers of AF [7]. The importance of a history, including modifiable risk factors, is imperative. Modifiable risk factors are those that can potentially be changed by using EB interventions and strategies; nonmodifiable risk factors are those which currently cannot be changed (Table 1). Research indicates that AF is strongly linked to acquired risk factors that positively react to health-prevention and health-promotion strategies [13].

A first-degree relative with AF increases the probability of a genetic predisposition to the arrhythmia [3]. A history of a metabolic disturbance or structural heart disease points to possible triggers for AF. Determination of the duration of the AF helps categorize the arrhythmia for treatment/management decisions. Because the pathogenesis of AF is often multifactorial, assessing for the relationship of AF with the pathophysiology of cardiovascular and thrombotic mechanisms, related to stroke risk, is also foundational [15].

For patients who present to the clinic with common complaints (overall fatigue, poor physical activity tolerance, generalized weakness, dizziness), review-of-systems questions should be mindful and targeted, based on specific patient characteristics (age, gender, race/ethnicity) and risk factors (eg, underlying cardiovascular disease, diabetes, thyroid conditions, vulnerability). There is no gold standard for review of systems [16]. Probing each individual patient symptom can be based on the mnemonic OLD CARTS, with the focus being person-centered:

Table 1
Modifiable and nonmodifiable risk factors for atrial fibrillation

Modifiable risk factors	Nonmodifiable risk factors
• Body mass index; per unit	• Age (increasing)
• Chronic (long-standing) use of alcohol	• Family history
• Diabetes (including prediabetes)	• Gender
• Elevated waist circumference	• Race/ethnicity
• Heart failure	
• Hyperlipidemia	
• Hypertension	
• Impaired fasting glucose	
• Lack of physical activity (sedentary lifestyle)	
• Left ventricular hypertrophy; reversible in some people	
• Low high-density lipoprotein cholesterol	
• Obesity	
• Obstructive sleep apnea	
• Overweight	
• Smoking (cigarettes)	

- Onset
- Location, radiation
- Duration
- Character
- Aggravating factors (what makes it worse); precipitating events (what causes onset)
- Relieving factors (what makes it better)
- Timing
- Severity
- What does the person think it is?

An additional question for older adults relates to any new medication, including vitamins, herbals, and supplements as well as prescribed, over-the-counter, and home remedies. A brown-bag approach (BBA) can be a helpful strategy. Wolff and colleagues [17] discovered that when the BBA was used, medication discrepancies decreased from 89% to 66%. The PCP simply asks the patient to bring in all of the medication remedies they have at home, in a brown bag. It is helpful to remember that the BBA alone is not sufficient unless it is paired with targeted questions [18]. The process is time consuming but does help the PCP understand the array of medications the older adult may be using at any time, some of which may contribute to the presence of AF.

Other areas to probe include asking the older adult about use of sleeping pills, alcohol, illicit drugs, or diet pills. Sleep/rest patterns and any recent acute illness help the PCP to better understand the patient's lifestyle.

Physical examination

The physical examination (PE) focuses on evidence of HF (pulmonary rales, S3 gallop, peripheral pulses, and jugular venous distention) as well as possible triggers. An irregularly irregular heart rate is present with auscultation. A variable intensity in the first heart sound may be present. The presence of a cardiac murmur requires further investigation for etiology (consider aortic or mitral stenosis). Blood pressure may be lower than baseline because of the decrease in atrial end-diastolic volume.

Physical findings of peripheral and/or abdominal edema, jugular venous distention, rales, and a third heart sound indicate the presence of HF. Any patient with signs of hemodynamic instability should be transferred to the emergency department for acute-care intervention.

Diagnostic testing

An ECG is key in the diagnosis of AF. It is the first test ordered in primary care to confirm history and PE findings. If the patient is experiencing only intermittent symptoms, ambulatory heart rhythm monitoring is used to define the arrhythmia. The duration of the monitoring can initially be determined by the frequency of the patient's symptoms. Event monitoring, either automatically activated or activated by the patient, is an option for patients with symptoms less than daily. A chest radiograph is ordered to evaluate causes or sequela of AF; radiography is an initial evaluation if pulmonary disease, HF, or cardiomegaly is suspected. Laboratory evaluation of electrolytes, a complete blood count, thyroid function, and renal and hepatic function are ordered to rule out systemic disease as the cause of the AF.

Additional testing may be necessary depending on the older adult's history and risk factors. Imaging studies include two-dimensional transthoracic echocardiography to evaluate cardiac structure and function [14]. Other tests may include:

- Stress echocardiography
- Nuclear perfusion imaging
- Cardiac catheterization (for evaluation of ischemia or coronary artery disease)
- Drug screening (selected cases)
- Sleep study (if sleep apnea is suspected)

Referral to a cardiologist is important for patients with complex cardiac disease and new-onset AF. A transthoracic echocardiogram or transesophageal echocardiogram is required to test for a left atrial thrombus, structural defects, and right and left heart function. In addition, testing for arterial disease via stress testing is necessary. Stress testing determines the extent of coronary artery disease [14].

TREATMENT

The goals of AF treatment and management are to (1) control heart rate, (2) prevent thromboembolic episodes, (3) improve QoL, and (4) reduce transitions of care across the spectrum. Prescribing anticoagulant therapy and rhythm or rate control are essential for these patients.

The treatment plan is determined by classification of the AF as well as the patient values and life goals. Patient outcomes from specific therapies are related to the duration and frequency of the AF. The role of nurse practitioners (NPs) in primary care is to collaborate with the older adult in shared decision making regarding treatment decisions. A holistic, patient-centered perspective helps the NP to integrate the patient's lifestyle and preferences into decision making.

Thromboembolism prevention

The approach to thromboembolism prevention is different in valvular and non-valvular AF. Evaluation of the patient by PE and with an echocardiogram assists in determining the AF. Valvular AF, caused by moderate to severe mitral stenosis or an artificial valve, requires long-term anticoagulation with warfarin [8]. Patients with other valvular disorders, such as communicant AF, should be treated on the basis of an analysis or risks and benefits. The patient's risk for thromboembolism and major bleeding from anticoagulant therapy is assessed using decision support tools. The patient is reassessed periodically to determine the need for a change in therapy.

The American Heart Association and American College of Cardiology guidelines on the treatment of AF recommend the use of the CHA_2DS_2-VASc scoring system for the assessment of stroke risk in patients with nonvalvular AF [8]. CHA$_2$DS$_2$-VASc is a mnemonic for the risk factors in the scoring tool. The tool can be downloaded to a smartphone device or accessed via computer on the Internet. The risk factors are weighed relative to the stroke risk. A personal history of stroke, transient ischemic attack, or thromboembolism carries a greater weight than having a previous myocardial infarction. A CHA$_2$DS$_2$-VASc score of 1 carries a 1.3% adjusted stroke rate per year while a score of 9 carries a 15.2% rate [8]. Oral anticoagulants are recommended in male patients with a CHA$_2$DS$_2$-VASc score of 2 or greater and female patients with a CHA$_2$DS$_2$-VASc score of 3 or greater [8]. For patients with a CHA$_2$DS$_2$-VASc score of 0 or 1, appropriate treatment options are no oral anticoagulant or aspirin.

Non–vitamin K oral anticoagulants (NOACs) are recommended for anticoagulant therapy. NOACs are preferred over oral warfarin because of the lower risk of life-threatening bleeding and no need for frequent monitoring of levels. However, NOACs have a significantly higher cost per month than warfarin. Patients with restricted prescription coverage may find the cost prohibitive. There are 2 types of NOACs, direct thrombin inhibitors and factor Xa inhibitors. The only direct thrombin inhibitor currently approved in the United States is dabigatran (Pradaxa). It has the benefit of having a reversal agent, idarucizumab (Praxbind), for management of patients undergoing procedures or experiencing bleeding. Factor Xa inhibitors include apixaban (Eliquis), edoxaban (Savaysa), and rivaroxaban (Xarelto) [19]. A reversal agent, coagulation factor Xa inactivated (Andexxa), is available for rivaroxaban and apixaban only. Particular attention to dosing is given in patients with impaired renal or hepatic function. NOACs should not be used in patients with end-stage renal or liver failure.

Warfarin is the recommended anticoagulant for patients with an artificial heart valve or moderate to severe mitral stenosis. However, it can also be used in patients for whom cost or other considerations prohibit NOAC use. The international normalized ratio (INR) should be measured at least weekly during start of therapy and at least monthly for ongoing monitoring [8]. The target INR level is generally set at 2.0 to 3.0. A decision regarding anticoagulant therapy includes shared decision making with the older adult regarding risks and benefits.

HAS-BLED is a risk-stratification tool for bleeding from anticoagulant therapy. HAS-BLED is paired with CHA$_2$DS$_2$-VASc scoring to assist in considering the risks and benefits of anticoagulant therapy. Table 2 lists the risk factors for bleeding and points assigned to each factor. Factors include:

- Systolic blood pressure greater than 160
- Abnormal liver or renal function
- A history of stroke or bleeding
- Labile INRs (if on warfarin)
- Age greater than 65 years
- Use of drugs that promote bleeding such as nonsteroidal anti-inflammatories or excessive alcohol intake [20].

Table 2 HAS-BLED scoring system	
Risk factors	Points
Hypertension: systolic blood pressure >160 mm Hg	1
Abnormal renal and liver function (1 point each)	1 or 2
Stroke	1
Bleeding tendency/predisposition	1
Labile INRs (if on warfarin)	1
Older adult (age >65 y)	1
Drug or alcohol (1 point each)	1 or 2
Maximum score	9

From Pisters R, Lane DA, Nieuwlaat R, de Vos CB, Crijns HJ, Lip GY. A novel user-friendly score (HAS-BLED) to assess one-year risk of major bleeding in atrial fibrillation patients: The Euro Heart Survey, Chest. 2010 Nov;138(5):1093-100. https://doi.org/10.1378/chest.10-0134. Epub 2010 Mar 18; with permission.

A score of 3 or greater is considered high risk for major bleeding. HAS-BLED is not recommended as a tool to exclude patients from use of anticoagulant therapy [20]. Rather, it is meant to focus on risk factors and the possibility of lowering risk by modifications in lifestyle or medical therapy.

Rate control

Control of ventricular rate is a priority for the patient with AF. Long-term tachycardia can result in cardiomyopathy and HF. Guidelines recommend the use of a β-blocker or nondihydropyridine calcium-channel blocker for rate control in all categories of AF [8]. Hemodynamically unstable patients should be transported to the emergency department for acute management with intravenous medications or direct current cardioversion. The target resting heart rate for patients with AF is individualized to the patient. Choice of medication, target heart rate, and medication dosing is based on the patient's comorbidities, symptom management, and shared decision making. An acceptable range for resting heart rate is 80 to 100 beats per minute.

β-Blockers are the most commonly used medications for rate control in AF [8]. β-Blockers block β-adrenergic receptors, thus lowering heart rate and the force of myocardial contraction. Oral formulations of metoprolol (tartrate or succinate), atenolol, esmolol, propranolol, nadolol, carvedilol, or bisoprolol can be used. β-Blockers should be slowly titrated to the target heart rate to avoid bradycardia. Patients with AF and HF may benefit from the use of carvedilol, which provides heart-rate control as well as improving left ventricular function. Patients should be monitored for side effects of the β-blocker as the medication is being titrated. Noncardiovascular side effects include fatigue, depression, insomnia, and bronchospasm [8].

An acceptable alternative to β-blockers are the nondihydropyridine calcium-channel blockers, verapamil or diltiazem. Nondihydropyridine calcium-channel blockers act to block the influx of calcium in the atrial-ventricular node, decreasing conduction of supraventricular impulses and decreasing heart rate. Both resting and exercise heart rate are reduced with nondihydropyridine calcium-channel blockers [8]. Caution is required when using verapamil or diltiazem in patients with HF: they are contraindicated in patients with a reduced left ventricular ejection fraction. As with β-blockers, nondihydropyridine calcium-channel blockers should be slowly titrated to minimize hypotension and bradycardia. Peripheral edema is common with both verapamil and diltiazem and may necessitate use of an alternative medication.

Digoxin is a second-line agent for rate control in AF. Atrial-ventricular node conduction is reduced by digoxin through a direct effect on sodium-potassium transport and vagal stimulation [21]. Digoxin reduces resting heart rate; it has no effect on rate during exercise [8]. Digoxin should be used with caution in older adults and in renal dysfunction because it can have toxic effects even at recommended doses. Serum levels of digoxin should be tested periodically. The optimal range is 0.5 to 1.0 ng/mL [21]. Increased morbidity and mortality is associated with levels greater than 1.0 ng/mL. Physical symptoms of digoxin toxicity include nausea and vomiting, confusion, and ventricular arrhythmias.

Amiodarone is a second-line agent for rate control in AF because it has the dual action of blocking calcium channels and blocking β-adrenergic receptors. Amiodarone reduces conduction of the fibrillatory waves through the atrial-ventricular node, thus slowing the ventricular heart rate. In its oral form, amiodarone is absorbed best with food. It has toxic effects on eyes, skin, liver, thyroid, nerves, and lungs. Long-term use is not recommended in most patients.

Rhythm control

Although rate control is the priority strategy for management of AF, patients may experience improved symptoms and QoL with conversion to NSR [8]. The strategy chosen, rate or rhythm control, is based on the hemodynamic status of the patient as well as consideration of patient preference and comorbidities. Patients with AF for less than 48 hours are the best candidates for the rhythm-control strategy. AF of longer duration results in remodeling of the myocardium, which changes both the electrical conduction pathways and myocardial muscle structure. The remodeling makes it more difficult to convert the rhythm. If cardioversion is chosen for patients with AF of greater than 48 hours' duration, warfarin or NOACs are recommended for at least 3 weeks before, and 4 weeks after cardioversion [8]. Anticoagulation is used before and after cardioversion regardless of the CHA_2DS_2-VASc score. A transesophageal echocardiogram is completed to detect left atrial thrombus before cardioversion. Rhythm control can be accomplished by direct current, medications, or catheter ablation.

Direct current cardioversion is used for emergency cardioversion as well as a rhythm-control strategy. Direct current shock is synchronized with the ventricular impulses to avoid ventricular fibrillation (Fig. 3). If the direct current shock fails to convert the rhythm, pad placement, energy waveform, and the amount of electrical energy are altered and another attempt is made. Pretreatment with antiarrhythmic medications may increase the probability of

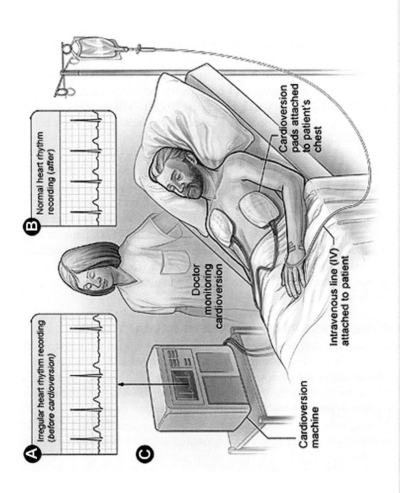

Fig. 3. Cardioversion procedure. (A) Rhythm before cardioversion. (B) Rhythm after cardioversion. (C) Defibrillator. (*From* Wikimedia Commons. Availabe at: https://commons.wikimedia.org/wiki/Category:Cardioversion#/media/File:Cardioversion.jpg. Accessed October 10, 2019.)

conversion to NSR in some patients. Success rates for direct current cardiover-sion are reported to be between 86% and 96% [22]. However, AF recurs in approximately 20% of patients overall and 40% of patients with HF, vascular disease, and recurrent AF, and who are older than 65 years. The complications of direct current cardioversion include thromboembolism, arrhythmias, muscle pain, and cutaneous burns [8].

Pharmacologic conversion is accomplished using a variety of antiarrhythmic medications. Medications used for pharmacologic cardioversion are amiodar-one, dofetilide, dronedarone, flecainide, propafenone, and sotalol [8]. The choice of medication is based on the patient's chronic comorbid conditions. Amiodarone is not recommended as a first-line agent because of its hepatic and renal toxicity. Dronedarone is not used in patients with HF. The choice of medications involves a discussion of risks versus benefits of antiarrhythmic medications in shared decision making with the patient. The primary care NP should be aware of the medication adverse reactions to facilitate the early detec-tion of complications and insure patient safety.

Catheter ablation cardioversion is an alternative strategy for conversion to sinus rhythm. Catheter ablation involves location of the abnormal fibrillatory foci and ablation of the tissue using radiofrequency or cryothermic destruction. The most abnormal foci are located at the ostia of the pulmonary veins. Catheter ablation is indicated in patients with symptomatic AF and HF with reduced ejection fraction [8]. AF recurs in approximately 20% of patients after catheter ablation [23]. In comparison with pharmacologic therapy, catheter ablation was found to lower hospitalization and death from HF. However, su-periority of this rhythm-control strategy is still controversial and requires addi-tional research.

ROLE OF THE NURSE PRACTITIONER IN PRIMARY CARE

The primary care NP can play an important part in the care of the patient with AF. Initial diagnosis of AF most often occurs in primary care. It is important for the NP to be aware of the symptoms of AF in older adults. Subtle symptoms such as lack of energy may be the only indicator of AF. The NP should pay special attention to patients with multiple risk factors.

Once the diagnosis of AF is established, the primary care NP has a role in helping the patient with decision making. Shared decision making is a factor in treatment decision [8,24]. The relationship established in primary care be-tween patient and clinician allows for the integration of patient preferences and comorbid conditions. Patients come to their primary care clinicians for advice and reassurance related to treatment choices. In addition, the primary care NP may be the first to be alerted to adverse reactions to medications or complications from procedures.

Finally, the primary care NP has a role as care manager for the patient with AF. Medication for thromboembolism prevention and rate or rhythm control are a small portion of the overall care of the patient. The primary care NP pro-vides periodic re-evaluation of the goals of therapy along with assessment of patient's needs and preferences. The holistic perspective of the primary care NP is invaluable for overall health and QoL in the older adult with AF.

Disclosure

The author has no commercial or financial conflicts of interest. No external source of funding was involved in writing this article.

References

[1] Centers for Disease Control and Prevention. Atrial fibrillation fact sheet. 2017. Available at: www.cdc.gov/dhdsp/data_statistics/fact_sheets/fs_atrial_fibrillation.htm. Accessed September 29, 2019.

[2] Chugh SS, Havmoeller R, Narayanan K, et al. Worldwide epidemiology of atrial fibrillation: a global burden of disease 2010 study. Circulation 2014;129(8):837–47.

[3] Lau DH, Nattel S, Kalman JM, et al. Modifiable risk factors and atrial fibrillation. Circulation 2017;136(6):583–96.

[4] Khaji A, Kowey PR. Update on atrial fibrillation. Trends Cardiovasc Med 2017;27(1): 14–25.

[5] Alagiakrishnan K, Banach M, Mah D, et al. Role of geriatric syndromes in the management of atrial fibrillation in older adults: a narrative review. J Am Med Dir Assoc 2019;20(2): 123–30.

[6] Medin J, Arbuckle R, Abetz L, et al. Development and validation of the AFSymp: an atrial fibrillation-specific measure of patient-reported symptoms. Patient 2014;7(3):319–27.

[7] Goldberger AL, Goldberger ZD, Shvilkin A. Clinical electrocardiography: a simplified approach. e-book. Philadelphia: Elsevier Health Sciences; 2017.

[8] January CT, Wann LS, Alpert JS, et al. 2014 AHA/ACC/HRS guideline for the management of patients with atrial fibrillation. J Am Coll Cardiol 2014;64(21):e1–76.

[9] Karamichalakis N, Letsas KP, Vlachos K, et al. Managing atrial fibrillation in the very elderly patient: challenges and solutions. Vasc Health Risk Manag 2015;11:555–62.

[10] National Heart, Lung, and Blood Institute. Atrial fibrillation. Available at: https://www.nhlbi.nih.gov/health-topics/atrial-fibrillation. Accessed October 11, 2019.

[11] Fabritz L, Guasch E, Antoniades C, et al. Defining the major health modifiers causing atrial fibrillation: a roadmap to underpin personalized prevention and treatment. Nat Rev Cardiol 2016;13(4):230–8.

[12] Fatkin D, Santiago CF, Huttner IG, et al. Genetics of atrial fibrillation: State of the art in 2017. Heart Lung Circ 2017;26(9):894–901.

[13] Wasmer K, Eckardt L, Breithardt G. Predisposing factors for atrial fibrillation in the elderly. J Geriatr Cardiol 2017;14(3):179–84.

[14] Gutierrez C, Blanchard D. Diagnosis and treatment of atrial fibrillation. Am Fam Physician 2016;94(6):442–52. Available at: https://www.aafp.org/afp/2016/0915/p442.pdf.

[15] Syed FF, Oral H. Editorial commentary: the holy grail of atrial fibrillation. Trends Cardiovasc Med 2017;1(27):26–8.

[16] Phillips A, Frank A, Loftin C, et al. A detailed review of systems: an educational feature. J Nurse Pract 2017;13(10):681–6.

[17] Wolff CM, Nowacki AS, Yeh J-Y, et al. A randomized controlled trial of two interventions to improve medication reconciliation. The Journal of the American Board of Family Medicine 2014;37(3):347–55.

[18] Sarzynski EM, Luz CC, Zhou S, et al. Medication reconciliation in an outpatient geriatrics clinic: does accuracy improve if patients "brown bag" their medications for appointments? J Amer Geriatr Soc 2014;62(3):567–9.

[19] Comparison of oral anticoagulants. Pharmacist's Letter/Prescriber's Letter 2018. Available at: https://prescriber.therapeuticresearch.com/Content/Segments/PRL/2016/May/Comparison-of-Oral-Anticoagulants-9673. Accessed October 11, 2019.

[20] Lane DA, Lip GYH. Use of the CHA2DS2-VASc and HAS-BLED scores to aid decision making for thromboprophylaxis in nonvalvular atrial fibrillation. Circulation 2012;126(7):860–5.

[21] Maury P, Rollin A, Galinier M, et al. Role of digoxin in controlling the ventricular rate during atrial fibrillation: a systematic review and a rethinking. Res Rep Clin Cardiol 2014;5: 93–101.

[22] Jaakkola S, Lip GYH, Biancari F, et al. Predicting unsuccessful electrical cardioversion for acute atrial fibrillation (from the AF-CVS Score). Am J Cardiol 2017;119(5):749–52.

[23] Marrouche NF, Brachmann J, Andresen D, et al. Catheter ablation for atrial fibrillation with heart failure. N Engl J Med 2018;378(5):417–27.

[24] January CT, Wann LS, Calkins H, et al. 2019 AHA/ACC/HRS focused update of the 2014 AHA/ACC/HRS guideline for the management of patients with atrial fibrillation: a report of the American College of Cardiology/American Heart Association Task Force on clinical practice guidelines and the Heart Rhythm Society in collaboration with the Society of Thoracic Surgeons. Circulation 2019;140(2):e125–51.

Advances in Family Practice Nursing 2 (2020) 63–75

ADVANCES IN FAMILY PRACTICE NURSING

Managing Older Adults with Type 2 Diabetes
Clinical Insights and Pearls

Denise Soltow Hershey, PhD, FNP-BC

College of Nursing, Michigan State University, 1355 Bogue Street, A127 Life Sciences, East Lansing, MI 48824, USA

Keywords
- Type 2 diabetes • Older adults • End of life • Diabetes management

Key points
- A1c target for older adults should be less than 8.0%.
- Use cautiously or avoid diabetes medications that increase risk for hypoglycemia in older adults.
- Be willing to deintensify and adjust medications as the individual ages to prevent adverse events, such as falls.
- Discuss and set mutual goals for diabetes management with the patient and his or her caregiver.

T ype 2 diabetes (T2D) is a common endocrine disorder that develops as individuals age. T2D occurs in 9% of adults, and in 20% of adults age 65 and older [1]. Aging in combination with diabetes, increases the risk of functional decline and disability in older adults [2]. Diabetes increases the risk for the development of frailty and muscle loss, which increases the risk for disability in this population [2]. Frailty and disability combined with the risk for hypoglycemia, in older adults with T2D, creates an environment for the increased incidence of falls and lower quality of life (QOL) [3]. Current guidelines for the management of T2D in older adults recommend less aggressive treatment and higher levels of hemoglobin A1c (A1c) for glycemic control to decrease the occurrence of hypoglycemic events [4]. This article discusses the current recommendations for the management of T2D in older adults across

E-mail address: soltowde@msu.edu

https://doi.org/10.1016/j.yfpn.2020.01.001
2589-420X/20/© 2020 Elsevier Inc. All rights reserved.

the trajectory from fit older adult to frail elder, and end-of-life treatment (EOL) considerations.

PATHOPHYSIOLOGY

Diabetes is a complex chronic condition, if undiagnosed and untreated, it can lead to the development of microvascular and macrovascular complications [5]. Diabetes is defined as a fasting plasma glucose $\geq$126 mg/dL or an A1c $\geq$6.5 [5]. Diabetes can be classified as either type 1 (autoimmune destruction of β-cells, leads to insulin deficiency) or type 2 (progressive loss of β-cell secretion due to insulin resistance) [5]. Type 1 diabetes is more likely to occur in younger adults, and was previously referred to as juvenile onset. As individuals with diabetes are living longer, health care providers may encounter older adults with type 1 diabetes [5,6].

Diabetes is prevalent in older adults; 90% to 95% of older adults with diabetes have T2D. The risk of diabetes increases as individuals age due to genetic, lifestyle, and aging influences. All of these factors contribute to the development of hyperglycemia (fasting plasma glucose [FPG] $\geq$126 mg/dL) [7]. This increased risk for hyperglycemia is associated with the development of insulin resistance and insulin secretion [7,8]. Accumulation of fat in the liver and muscles, as well as a decrease in mitochondrial activity in the brain and muscles, contributes to the development of insulin resistance [8]. Impairment of β-cell function related to aging negatively influences insulin secretion [7,8] (Fig. 1).

The criteria for diagnosing diabetes in older adults is the same as that for all other adults. Diabetes can be asymptomatic, and diagnoses is usually made through routine laboratory tests. Older adults may present differently from individuals of younger age. These differences include dehydration, confusion, incontinence, and diabetes complications, such as neuropathy or nephropathy [7,8].

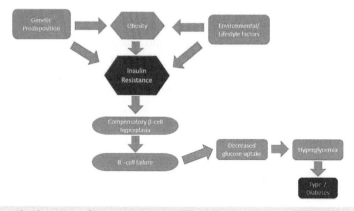

Fig. 1. Pathophysiology of type 2 diabetes development.

The pathophysiological changes identified previously increase the risk for the development of hyperglycemia. Older adults with T2D are at increased risk for hypoglycemia (FPG ≤70 mg/dL) as well [9]. These risk factors include the following:

- Medications used in the treatment of T2D
- Psychosocial factors, such as living alone, reduced food intake, and depression
- Cognitive issues of memory loss and dementia; sensory changes of hearing loss and diminished taste
- Motor changes associated with decreased dexterity, reduced physical activity, and impaired mobility
- Comorbidities
- Decreased renal and hepatic function
- An overall decreased awareness of the symptoms associated with hypoglycemia [10]

Hypoglycemia frequently occurs in older adults who are receiving intensive glycemic control. Management guidelines do recommend different ranges for glycemic control based on where the older adult falls within the aging trajectory (management is discussed in a later section).

DIAGNOSIS AND GLYCEMIC TARGETS

Screening and diagnostic recommendations for older adults are not different than for younger ages. The American Diabetes Association (ADA) 2019 guidelines recommend screening for diabetes every 3 years in individuals age 45 or older. Screening that is more frequent is encouraged in those who are at higher risk. Factors that increase risk are older age (particularly those older than 60), male sex, history of gestational diabetes, family history (particularly mother, father, or sibling), comorbidity of hypertension and obesity, and inactive lifestyle. Patients with 1 or more of these risk factors should be screened at more frequent intervals [5]. Fasting plasma glucose, a 2-hour oral glucose tolerance test, or an A1c, can be used to screen for prediabetes (A1c <6.5%) and diabetes in older adults (see Table 1 for diagnostic criteria).

Diagnostic criteria for diabetes do not change as individuals age, the recommendations for level of glycemic control in older adults can vary based on age and health status. The overall A1c goal for adults is an A1c <7%, for adults who are higher risk for hypoglycemia, limited life expectancy, and comorbid

Table 1
Diagnostic criteria for prediabetes and diabetes

Diagnostic test	Prediabetes	Diabetes
Oral glucose tolerance test 2-h post	140–199 mg/dL	≥200 mg/dL
Fasting plasma glucose	100–125 mg/dL	≥126 mg/dL
A1c	5.7%–6.4%	≥6.5%

Data from American Diabetes Association. 2. Classification and Diagnosis of Diabetes: Standards of Medical Care in Diabetes-2019. Diabetes Care. 2019 Jan;42(Suppl 1): S13-S28. https://doi.org/10.2337/dc19-S002.

conditions a less stringent A1c goal of <8% may be more appropriate [9]. Tight glycemic control in older adults has been associated with greater risk and occurrence of hypoglycemia [4]. Spain and Edlund [11] identified that A1c values in the mid-range of 6% to 8% may be more beneficial over time than lower values in older adults. A1c targets for older adults should be based on their overall health status. For the fit older adult, a target of 7.5% is reasonable, for those with moderate to severe frailty 8.0% should be the goal, and for the very severe frail 8.5% should be the goal [2].

MANAGEMENT OF TYPE 2 DIABETES

The management of T2D in older adults varies based on the overall health status of the patient. Individualization of treatment is essential. Goals for treatment need to be based on functional status, risk for hypoglycemia, prevention of hospital admissions, and the maintenance and/or improvement of functional status [2]. For the fit or high-functioning older adult, management of T2D is similar to that of younger adults [2,12]. As functioning and health decline, individualization of management increases and becomes more collaborative between primary care, specialist, home care, long-term care, and hospital settings [2,6,12]. Along with the management of diabetes, the prevention and/or management of other comorbidities, such as hypertension (HTN), hyperlipidemia, and obesity need to be incorporated into the plan of care. One of the main goals in diabetes management in older adults is the prevention of hypoglycemia.

Hypoglycemia in older adults has been associated with an increased risk for heart failure (HF), dementia, myocardial infarction (MI), stroke, fall, fractures, and death [13]. The prevention of hypoglycemia includes allowing for less strict levels of glycemic control, and the avoidance, if possible, of medications that have a higher risk of producing hypoglycemia [13]. Sulfonylureas and insulins are the 2 classes of glycemic-lowering agents that are at higher risk for causing hypoglycemia [8,11,14].

When considering medications for the older adult with T2D, the one-size-fit all approach is not appropriate. Unless initiation of medications is low and the patient is monitored closely, the older adult may develop or experience an exacerbation of geriatric syndromes and increased disease burden [11]. The use of sulfonylureas should be done with caution. Sulfonylureas not only increase the risk for hypoglycemia, but also the risk for falls. Rajpathak and colleagues [15] found older adults on sulfonylureas had an increased risk of incurring a hip fracture, due to hypoglycemic-related [15]. Metformin, linagliptin, sitagliptin, GLP-1 receptor agonists, and sodium-glucose cotransporter 2 inhibitors have been found to have a lower risk of hypoglycemia and are preferred agents in the treatment of T2D in older adults [14].

MEDICATION SELECTION

Metformin is the recommend first-line medication for older adults who do not have a contraindication. Most older adults will require more than one medication as their disease progresses. The selection of a second-agent option includes the use of sulfonylureas, DPP-4 inhibitors, or SGLT2 inhibitors. Sulfonylureas should be used with caution because of their increased risk for hypoglycemia. If glycemic targets are not achieved, the addition of an insulin would be appropriate. It is not uncommon for adults to be on 2 to 3 different agents before the introduction of insulin. If a patient is already on a sulfonylurea, as insulin is introduced, the sulfonylurea should be tapered and discontinued due to the increased risk of hypoglycemia that can occur with the combination of these medications [7,16]. Table 2 provides an overview of glycemic-lowering agents, their adverse effects, impact on A1c level, and considerations with regard to their use in older adults.

INAPPROPRIATE POLYPHARMACY

Older adults with diabetes are at high risk for inappropriate polypharmacy, related to the potential need for the use of multiple antidiabetic medications to maintain glycemic control, and the fact they may be on multiple medications to manage other comorbidities [7,8,17]. One goal of management should be the minimization of inappropriate polypharmacy in this population. Health care providers (HCPs) need to consider if intensifying treatment is necessary. Factors that should be considered are as follows: (1) Can other medications be reduced or eliminated as new medications are added? (2) What adverse effects need to be considered, hypoglycemia, weight gain, edema, HF, and gastrointestinal effects? Will some of these effects be increased by the addition of a new medication? If so, consider stopping the medication most likely to contribute to the development of the adverse effects. (3) What are the patient's preferences? (4) What is the patient's and caregiver's capacity? Are they capable and do they have the functional and cognitive capacity to follow the prescribed plan and monitor for potential adverse effects [8]?

As HCPs, it is important to assess the patient's ability to follow medication regimens; as additional medications are added, assess for interactions between medications and side effects [17]. Inappropriate polypharmacy increases the risk for side effects and drug interactions, there are times that either simplification and or deintensification of a regimen should be considered [17]. The ADA 2019 [6] recommendations for simplification, deprescribing/deintensification can be found in Table 3.

MANAGEMENT OF COMORBIDITIES

Management of lifestyle factors to prevent and reduce risks associated with hyperlipidemia, heart disease, obesity, and frailty are important in the older adult with T2D. The risk of morbidity and mortality is significantly lowered when cardiovascular (CV) risk factors are managed and controlled [6]. Effective diabetes management not only includes the control of glucose levels, but also management of lipids and blood pressure, to minimize both macrovascular and microvascular complications associated with diabetes [11].

Table 2
Overview of glycemic-lowering agents with considerations for use in older adults with type 2 diabetes

Agent	Route of administration	Dosing	A1c reduction	Adverse effects	Considerations for use in older adults
Biguanides Metformin	Oral	850–1000 mg BID	1%–2%	• GI effects (N/D) are common (can be dosage related)	• Recommended initial therapy • Low risk of hypoglycemia • Reduce cardiovascular events and mortality • Do not use if eGFR (estimated glomerular filtration rate) < 30 • Avoid in patients with decompensated HF
Sulfonylureas Glyburide Glipizide Glimepiride	Oral	1.25–20 mg daily 2.5–20 mg daily 1–4 mg daily	1%–2%	• Risk of hypoglycemia • Weight gain • Increased risk of CV mortality	• Use with caution • Glyburide not recommended • Glipizide and glimepiride need to be used very cautiously
Thiazolidinediones Pioglitazone Rosiglitazone	Oral	15–45 mg daily 4–8 mg daily	1%–2%	• Fluid retention • Weight gain • Fracture risk • Bladder cancer (pioglitazone) • Increased LDL (rosiglitazone) • Increased risk for MI (rosiglitazone)	• Do not use in patients with renal impairment • Use cautiously in hepatic insufficiency, HF, and coronary artery disease • Avoid in patients who are a fall risk or at high risk for fractures

Drug class / Medication	Route	Dose	A1c reduction	Side effects	Considerations
α-Glucosidase inhibitors Acarbose	Oral	50–100 mg TID	0.4%–0.9%	• Flatulence • Diarrhea • Abdominal pain	• CV events decreased in patients with impaired glucose tolerance • Do not use in patients with comorbid liver or bowel disease or if serum creatinine > 2 mg/dL
Meglitinides Repaglinide nateglinide	Oral	0.5–4 mg before each meal 60–120 mg TID before meals	0.4%–0.9%	• Weight gain • Peripheral edema • Hepatotoxicity • GI disturbances • Risk of hypoglycemia	• Avoid in renal dysfunction • Hypoglycemic effect enhanced by gemfibrozil
Amylin mimetics Pramlintide	Subcutaneous injection	120 μg before meals		• N/V • Risk of hypoglycemia when used with insulin	• Should not be used in patients with an A1c >9% • Avoid use in patients with decreased hypoglycemia awareness • Avoid in patients with history of poor adherence
GLP-1 receptor agonist Exenatide Liraglutide Lixisenatide	Subcutaneous injection	5–10 μg BID 1.2–1.8 mg daily 20 μg daily	1%–1.5%	• Weight loss • N/V/Diarrhea • Risk for acute pancreatitis • Injection site reactions • Increased risk of hypoglycemia when taking sulfonylureas	• Increased risk of side effects in patients with renal insufficiency • Exenatide not indicated with eGFR <30 • Caution when using lixisenatide • Liraglutide may provide some CV benefits • Good motor skills and visual acuity needed due to being an injectable

(continued on next page)

Table 2
(continued)

Agent	Route of administration	Dosing	A1c reduction	Adverse effects	Considerations for use in older adults
DPP-4 inhibitors Sitagliptin Saxagliptin Linagliptin Alogliptin	Oral	100 mg daily 2.5–5.0 mg daily 5 mg daily 25 mg daily	0.5%–0.8%	• Joint pain • Skin lesions • Potential risk of acute pancreatitis	• Can be used in renal impairment • Renal dose adjustment required for linagliptin
SGLT2 inhibitors Dapagliflozin Canagliflozin Empagliflozin	Oral	5–10 mg daily 100–300 mg daily 10–25 mg daily	0.5%–0.7%	• Weight loss • Blood pressure lowering • Vulvovaginal candidiasis • Urinary tract infection • Risk of euglycemic diabetic ketoacidosis • Risk of amputation and fractures with canagliflozin • Increased LDL cholesterol	• May lead to abnormalities in renal function • Avoid in older patients with preexisting renal impairment • Avoid when eGFR <60
Insulin Novolog Humalog [7,8,17]	Subcutaneous injection	Individualized	No limit	• Hypoglycemia • Weight gain	• Dosing errors can occur with functional and cognitive changes in older adults • Can challenge self-management capacity • Lower doses may be required in patients with lower eGFR

| Lantus (insulin glargine) | Subcutaneous injection | Individualized | No limit | • Hypoglycemia
• Weight gain
• Peripheral edema | • Caution in renal or hepatic impairment
• Caution with visual impairment |

Abbreviations: BID, twice a day; CV, cardiovascular; eGFR, estimated glomerular filtration rate; GI, gastrointestinal; HF, heart failure; LDL, low-density lipoprotein; MI, myocardial infarction; N/V, nausea/vomiting; TID, 3 times a day.
Data from Refs [8,11,14].

Table 3
American Diabetes Association 2019 recommendations for deintensification and simplification of treatment regimens in older adults with type 2 diabetes

Patient health status	Simplification	Deintensification/deprescribing
Healthy (few comorbidities, functional and cognitive status intact)	• Severe or recurrent hypoglycemia (if on insulin) • Wide glucose excursions • Decline in cognitive or functional status	• Severe or recurrent hypoglycemia on non-insulin therapy • Wide glucose excursions • Inappropriate polypharmacy is present
Complex/Intermediate (multiple comorbidities, 2 + instrumental ADL impairment or mild to moderate cognitive impairment)	• Severe or recurrent hypoglycemia (if on insulin) • Unable to manage complexity of insulin regimen • Significant change in social circumstances (loss of caregiver, financial difficulties, change in living situation)	• Severe or recurrent hypoglycemia on non-insulin therapy • Wide glucose excursions • Inappropriate polypharmacy is present
Community-dwelling (receiving care in a skilled nursing facility for ST rehabilitation)	• If treatment regimen was escalated during recent hospitalization, the reinstating of pre-hospital regimen is appropriate during rehabilitation	• If hospitalization resulted in weight loss, anorexia, ST cognitive decline, and/or loss of physical functioning
Very complex/poor health (LT care, end-stage chronic disease, moderate to severe cognitive impairment or 2 + ADL dependencies) EOL	• On insulin and patient desires to decrease number of injections and finger sticks • Inconsistent eating pattern • Pain or discomfort caused by treatment • Excessive caregiver stress due to treatment complexity	• On hypoglycemic agents with high risk of hypoglycemic events • Taking medications without clear benefit • Taking medications that do not have any clear benefit of improving symptoms and/or comfort

Abbreviations: ADL, activities of daily living; EOL, end of life; LT, long term; ST, short term.

Adapted from American Diabetes Association. 2. Classification and Diagnosis of Diabetes: Standards of Medical Care in Diabetes-2019.Diabetes Care. 2019 Jan;42(Suppl 1): S13-S28. htps://doi.org/10.2337/dc19-S002; with permission.

The monitoring and assessment of nutritional status in older adults with diabetes is important to decrease the risk of frailty and functional status decline. Eighty percent to 90% of patients with T2D are obese; in fit older patients, weight loss may be beneficial [2]. Older adults should be counseled regarding the importance of maintaining optimal nutrition, including adequate protein intake and to participate in regular aerobic and strength-training activities [6].

HTN and hyperlipidemia management in older adults with T2D has been found to be beneficial in lowering the risk for the development of CV complications (MI, stroke, CV death) [12]. In older adults with T2D, a target systolic blood pressure of approximately 140 mm Hg should be the goal. Having a systolic lower than 130 mm Hg has few benefits, and increases the risk for adverse events, falls, cognitive dysfunction, and frailty [12,18]. Lower blood pressure values may be related to chronic tissue hypoperfusion and secondary long-term damage contributing to the development of associated adverse effects [18]. Blood pressure targets and management should be part of a shared decision-making approach, and based on the patient's level of function. For frail individuals, blood pressure goals are more relaxed, with a target of 145 to 160/90 mm Hg [12].

Studies have shown that older individuals may benefit more from cholesterol management than younger adults. Hyperlipidemia should be managed in older adults withT2D up to the age of 80, with some studies showing benefit of cholesterol management through age 85 [12]. Statins are the recommended class of medications for the management of hyperlipidemia in older adults. For the older adult with severe morbidity, and/or limited life expectancy it is not recommended to start statins, and the removal of them should be considered [12,18]. The use of fibrates can be used on the healthy independent older adult, but are not recommended in the older adult who has severe frailty [12].

END OF LIFE

The goals of diabetes management at the EOL focus on decreasing symptoms and improving comfort [19–22]. One of the main treatment goals related to diabetes at the EOL needs to focus on the prevention of hypoglycemic and hyperosmolar hyperglycemic events (polydipsia and polyuria) [19,20,23]. During the EOL period, discussions around the management of diabetes is an essential component of the plan of care. Discussions need to center around frequency of glucose testing, continuation or stoppage of medication, and monitoring of glycemic control [19,20,23].

The management of diabetes will change as the patient approaches the EOL. Patients who have weeks to months to live should maintain glucose levels between 180 and 360 mg/dL [19,20,23]. Target levels are tailored based on the patient's preferences and risk for the development of hyperosmolar hyperglycemic events [19,20,23]. Requirements for self–blood glucose monitoring can be reduced from daily to every 3 days for patients with T2D and A1c's are no longer required [20,23]. Medications, oral and insulin, may need to be adjusted based on the patient's symptoms and risk for hyperosmolar glycemic events [19,20,23].

As the patient approaches the EOL, and has only days to live, and organ failure advances, the prevention of hypoglycemia is the main goal. Oral medications can be stopped, and glucose monitoring needs to be done only if the patient is exhibiting symptoms of hypoglycemia or hyperglycemia. For conscious patients who are experiencing hyperglycemic events, the use of short-acting insulin is appropriate [24].

The most essential component of care during this period is communication with the patient and family members. The patient and the family may find it uncomfortable with changes to a self-care regimen, and some members of the family may be reluctant to make the recommended changes [20]. Open communication with the patient and family needs to focus on the development of goals related to diabetes management and what to expect during the EOL period [19].

IMPLICATIONS FOR CLINICAL PRACTICE

Managing the older adult with T2D can be challenging for HCPs. Management plans need to take into consideration the patient's functional and cognitive status, as well as mutual preferences and values. For the older adult with T2D, management plans need to be collaboratively developed with the patient, including shared decision-making and mutual goal setting. Goals need to consider the patient's current functional status, prevention of hypoglycemia, and prevention of unnecessary hospital admissions. In addition, the goals should focus on improving the patient's functional health, and the reductions of disability while using the best possible resources [2]. Goals and changes to the plan of care will need to be adjusted as patients move across the aging trajectory from fit or healthy elder to EOL. HCPs need to be aware of and willing to make changes to the patient's plan of care to prevent hypoglycemia and its associated complications.

Disclosure
None.

References
[1] Schlender L, Martinez YV, Adeniji C, et al. Efficacy and safety of metformin in the management of type 2 diabetes mellitus in older adults: a systematic review for the development of recommendations to reduce potentially inappropriate prescribing. BMC Geriatr 2017;17(Suppl 1):99–117.

[2] Strain WD, Hope SV, Green A, et al. Type 2 diabetes mellitus in older people: a brief statement of key principles of modern day management including the assessment of frailty. A national collaborative stakeholder initiative. Diabet Med 2018;35(7):838–45.

[3] Chiba Y, Kimbara Y, Kodera R, et al. Risk factors associated with falls in elderly patients with type 2 diabetes. J Diabetes Complications 2015;29(7):898–902.

[4] Rodriguez Poncelas A, Barrot de la Puente J, Coll de Tuero G, et al. Glycaemic control and treatment of type 2 diabetes in adults aged 75 years or older. Int J Clin Pract 2018;72(3):1.

[5] ADA. Classification and diagnosis of diabetes: standards of medical care in diabetes - 2019. Diabetes Care 2019;32(1):S13–28.

[6] ADA. Older adults: standards of medical care in diabetes 2019. Diabetes Care 2019;42(supplement 1):S139–47.

[7] Lee PG, Halter JB. The pathophysiology of hyperglycemia in older adults: clinical considerations. Diabetes Care 2017;40(4):444–52.

[8] Lipska KJ, Krumholz H, Soones T, et al. Polypharmacy in the aging patient: a review of glycemic control in older adults with type 2 diabetes. JAMA 2016;315(10):1034–45.

[9] ADA. Glycemic targets: standards of medical care in diabetes - 2019. Diabetes Care 2019;42(Supplement 1):S61–70.

[10] Ballin MC. Hypoglycemia: a serious complication for the older adult with diabetes. Am J Nurs 2016;116(2):34–40.

[11] Spain M, Edlund BJ. Pharmacological management of type 2 diabetes in newly diagnosed older adults. J Gerontol Nurs 2009;35(7):16–21.

[12] Sinclair AJ, Abdelhafiz AH, Forbes A, et al. Evidence-based diabetes care for older people with Type 2 diabetes: a critical review. Diabet Med 2019;36(4):399–413.

[13] Arnold SV, Lipska KJ, Wang J, et al. Use of intensive glycemic management in older adults with diabetes mellitus. J Am Geriatr Soc 2018;66(6):1190–4.

[14] Freeman J. Management of hypoglycemia in older adults with type 2 diabetes. Postgrad Med 2019;131(4):241–50.

[15] Rajpathak S, Fu C, Brodovicz K, et al. Sulfonylurea use and risk of hip fractures among elderly men and women with type 2 diabetes. Drugs Aging 2015;32(4):321–7.

[16] ADA. Pharmacologic approaches to glycemic treatment: standards of medical care in diabetes 2019. Diabetes Care 2019;42(Supplement 1):S90–102.

[17] Bigelow A, Freeland B. Type 2 diabetes care in the elderly. J Nurse Pract 2017;13(3):181–8.

[18] Tessier DM, Meneilly GS, Moleski L, et al. Influence of blood pressure and other clinical variables on long-term mortality in a cohort of elderly subjects with type 2 diabetes. Can J Diabetes 2016;40(1):12–6.

[19] Jeffereys E, Rosielle D. Diabetes management at the end of life. J Palliat Med 2012;15:1142–54.

[20] King E, Haboubi H, Evans D, et al. The management of diabetes in terminal illness related to cancer. QJM 2012;105:3–9.

[21] Kondo S, Kondo M, Kondo A. Glycemic control using A1C level in terminal cancer patients with preexisting type 2 diabetes. J Palliat Med 2013;16:790–3.

[22] Quinn K, Hudson P, Dunning T. Diabetes management in patients receiving palliative care. J Pain Symptom Manage 2006;32:275–86.

[23] Angelo M, Ruchaiski C, Sproge B. An approach to diabetes mellitus in hospice and palliative medicine. J Palliat Med 2011;14:83–7.

[24] McCoubrie R, Jeffrey D, Paton C, et al. Managing diabetes mellitus in patients with advanced cancer: a case note audit and guidelines. Eur J Cancer Care 2005;14:244–8.

Women's Health

Advances in Family Practice Nursing 2 (2020) 77–85

ADVANCES IN FAMILY PRACTICE NURSING

ELSEVIER
MOSBY

Sexual Violence Screening for Women Across the Lifespan

Ginny Moore, DNP, WHNP-BC*,
Shaunna Parker, MSN, WHNP-BC,
Shelza Rivas, DNP, WHNP-BC, AGPCNP-BC,
Stefani Elizabeth Yudasz, DNP, WHNP-BC[1]

Vanderbilt University School of Nursing, 461 21st Avenue South, Godchaux Hall, Nashville, TN 37240, USA

Keywords

• Sexual violence • Screening methods • Women's health

Key points

- The incidence of sexual violence against women in the United States remains unconscionably high.
- Sexual violence has been identified as a serious public health issue affecting millions of women.
- Screening for sexual violence is a foundational step to intervention.
- Health care providers should be aware of sexual violence screening recommendations across the lifespan and use appropriate screening methods for adolescent, childbearing, and senior women.

O ne in 6 women in the United States will experience some form of sexual violence in her lifetime [1]. The violence may be in the form of intimate partner violence (IPV), which is also known as domestic or dating violence, reproductive coercion, sexual assault, and rape. Rape is a legal term defined specifically by each state. Typically, it includes the act of penetration. Sexual assault is also defined by each state but serves as a broader term encompassing sexual acts other than penetration. Reproductive coercion involves manipulation of one's reproductive decision making.

[1]Present address: 11050 Parkview Circle Drive. Fort Wayne. IN 46845.

*Corresponding author. E-mail address: ginny.moore@vanderbilt.edu

https://doi.org/10.1016/j.yfpn.2020.01.002
2589-420X/20/© 2020 Elsevier Inc. All rights reserved.

National statistics indicate a decline in rates of sexual violence, but the life-time incidence is still unconscionably high [1]. Sexual violence is a pervasive crime with potentially profound effects on victims. To minimize the effects, it is essential that health care providers identify women whose lives are affected by sexual violence. This article discusses the incidence of sexual violence across the women's health lifespan, reviews recommendations for sexual violence screening, and identifies screening methods appropriate for use in adolescent, childbearing, and senior populations.

ADOLESCENCE

Age ranges for adolescence vary among different professional organizations, but all agree that it is the transitional period between childhood and adulthood. Adolescent and young adult women are more likely to be victims of sexual as-sault than are women in all other age groups. Adolescent dating violence may take place in person or electronically in the form of repeated texting or the post-ing of sexual pictures online without consent. A survey revealed that 26% of women experienced IPV for the first time before 18 years [2,3].

Data suggest that IPV is most prevalent in adolescence and young adulthood and then begins to decline with age [2,3]. In addition, the earlier the exposure to IPV occurs, the more likely it is for adolescent girls to experience IPV. Early exposure, such as a childhood history of violence between parents, experiences of poor parenting, and child abuse and neglect, including sexual violence, all increase the risk of occurrence during the adolescent period [2,4]. The ease of accessibility to others through social media channels also presents challenges. Through these exchanges, adolescents meet strangers, develop trusting rela-tionships with the perpetrator, and allow themselves to be photographed nude or in sexually explicit poses. These acts often have a higher risk of leading to other forms of sexual exploitation and sexual assault. Misperceptions, atti-tudes regarding sexual assault, and the psychological trauma that accompanies these acts prevent adolescents from seeking medical care [4].

Recommendations from professional organizations lack consistency regarding when and how the screening is performed. Data suggest that resources and tools used within many communities are ineffective in identifying at-risk groups [5]. Regardless of differing opinions, all recommend routine screening and agree that adolescent screening provides the benefit of overcoming barriers to IPV disclosure. The American College of Obstetricians and Gynecologists (ACOG) recommends screening women and adolescent girls for reproductive and sexual coercion in a safe and supportive environment that respects confiden-tiality [5,6]. In addition, the American Academy of Pediatrics guidelines indicate screening for sexual victimization as a part of visits for psychosocial problems, sexuality issues, contraception or substance abuse, and health supervision [5].

During the adolescent period, many times there is a lack of information, un-derstanding, and knowledge about sexual violence. Because of this, health care providers have a responsibility to remain well informed and aware of the cogni-tive developmental differences between younger and older adolescents. Having an understanding of these differences plays a critical role in identifying how questions will be asked during visits. The Home, Education/Employment, Activities, Drugs, Sexuality, and Suicide/Depression (H.E.A.D.S.S) psychosocial assessment tool is used with high school and college aged students and guides questions by focusing on each of the areas listed in the tool's title [4]. In 2004, the H.E.A.D.S.S. assessment was expanded to H.E.E.A.D.S.S.S. to include questions about eating and safety. The newer version includes approximately 115 questions and emphasizes a strengths-based approach to the adolescent interview to foster patient-provider rapport and successful interventions [7]. Both versions of the assessment tool are readily accessible online with no associated cost.

Specifically inquiring about sexual history allows the health care provider an opportunity to obtain information concerning the first sexual experience, use of social media to find sexual partners, and a history of unwanted or forced sexual behaviors [4]. In addition, a discussion about previous alcohol and recreational drug use should be included. Health care providers must be aware that adolescents might be reluctant to report an incidence due to feelings of shame, guilt, and embarrassment [4]. It is recommended that providers facilitate disclosure by establishing environments that feel safe and welcoming. This includes the availability of educational materials, such as pamphlets and posters, and trained staff to address disclosure of the experiences [5]. In addition, it is important to discuss the limits of confidentiality and already have a referral plan in place. The adolescent patient should have a complete understanding that although they might not agree with the plan, reportable incidences are mandatory and must be reported.

The adolescent period is one in which growth and development take place. In addition, it is also when acceptance from others, self-identity, and discovering independence are most important. Adolescence is an impressionable period and is an ideal time for health care providers, parents/guardians, and other support persons to provide anticipatory guidance. Education on healthy behaviors, attitudes, and relationships is critical and influences how one might respond within future relationships.

CHILDBEARING YEARS

Childbearing years are defined by several professional organizations as the ages between 14 and 46 years [8,9]. Women of childbearing age, specifically pregnant women, are at increased risk of IPV, sexual assault, and rape [10]. The data demonstrate that approximately 43.6% of women in the United States have experienced some form of sexual violence [11]. A higher prevalence of rape occurs in minority women, with American Indian and Alaskan Native women residing on reservations being most at risk for rape [10]. Sexual assault on college campuses has also risen. A recent study showed that 1 in 4 heterosexual women experience sexual assault in the 4 years they spend in college, with bisexual and minority college women being most susceptible to sexual assault [12].

Pregnant women are especially vulnerable to IPV. Data demonstrate that IPV affects up to 22% of pregnant women and results in the delay of perinatal care [13]. In addition, IPV has been correlated to poor health outcomes for both mother and baby, including maternal and fetal death [13–15]. Most at risk of IPV are pregnant women who are younger in age with lower socioeconomic status, who are unmarried, have housing instability, and who have fewer years of education [14]. Ongoing fear and frequent threats caused by IPV correlate to significant mental health impairment that often results in post-traumatic stress disorder, major depressive disorder, anxiety, and substance abuse which persists through the postpartum period [13–15].

Often mothers are unable to appropriately bond with their baby after delivery and have difficulty breastfeeding as a result of IPV [14,15]. Obstetric complications are also strongly linked to IPV exposure. Vaginal bleeding, high blood pressure, severe nausea or vomiting, premature rupture of membranes and premature birth are among several complications [14]. A recent study showed that pregnant women who experience IPV are 5 times more likely to experience placental abruption and intrauterine fetal demise [14].

The perinatal period is a crucial opportunity for health care providers to screen and identify pregnant women experiencing IPV [13]. The nature of frequent visits during this period allows health care providers to be especially attentive to emotional and physical signs and symptoms [13]. Perinatal care may be the only type of health care that some women receive and many pregnant women present at this time with more barriers to leaving their partners [13]. Professional organizations have not recommended specific sexual violence screening tools for pregnant women, but ACOG continues to recommend regular screening intervals throughout the perinatal and postpartum periods [16].

Professional organizations have various perspectives regarding universal screening for sexual violence. General recommendations have concluded that health care providers should be routinely screening for sexual violence in all women, especially during initial and annual health care visits [9]. Women with a history of sexual violence, unemployment, substance abuse, and low socioeconomic status are at particularly increased risk of IPV and should be screened more frequently [9,17,18]. Similarly, childbearing women who report certain symptoms, such as depression, unexplained injuries, unexplained headaches, pelvic or abdominal pain, dysmenorrhea, and sexual dysfunction, should also be screened [9,17,18]. Although current recommendations have not established clear screening intervals for nonpregnant women, sexual violence screening should be performed at regular intervals for pregnant women during the perinatal period [9,13,16]. Pregnant women should be screened at the first prenatal visit, at least once per trimester, and at the postpartum visit [9,13,16].

Health care providers should be diligent about screening for sexual violence in all women during their reproductive years. Several verbal and written methods are available based on the patient's age, literacy level, language, and risk factors. ACOG recommend the SAVE Model Protocol as an approach to screening that includes (1) screening all patients for sexual violence, (2) asking direct questions in a nonjudgmental way, (3) validating the patient, and (4) evaluating, educating, and referring regardless of the method used [18].

The US Preventive Services Task Force recommends several well-studied screening tools that assess safety, physical abuse, emotional and physical IPV, as well as the frequency of sexual violence [19]. Humiliation, Afraid, Rape, Kick is a 4-item questionnaire that assesses for IPV within the past year [20]. Hurt, Insult, Threaten, Scream (HITS) is also a 4-item tool scored on a 5-point scale that assesses the frequency of IPV and is conducted through self-report or by a provider [21]. The extended version, E-HITS, specifically assesses the frequency of sexual violence [17]. The Partner Violence Screen is a 3-question tool that assesses for physical IPV and safety within the last year as well as current safety [21]. This particular tool is administered in urgent and emergency care settings by providers [20]. Finally, Woman Abuse Screening Tool is an 8-question survey that assesses physical and emotional IPV solely through self-report [21].

The long-term effects of sexual violence in women of childbearing age are significant. Survivors often experience decreased quality of life, mental health conditions, and chronic physical symptoms. Early intervention through screening has the potential to decrease the incidence of IPV and prevent these poor health outcomes in patients experiencing sexual violence.

SENIOR POPULATIONS

The definition of senior or elder varies, with the age of 60 to 65 years being the range for the beginning of this phase of life. Elder abuse is defined as "behavior by someone with an ongoing relationship to an elder, and a duty towards that elder, that may constitute: Willful infliction of physical pain or injury or unnecessary restraint (physical abuse), willful nonconsensual sexual contact (sexual abuse), or willful infliction of emotional harm (psychological abuse)." [22].

Although the incidence of sexual violence is higher in adolescence or childbearing years, it is important to remember that sexual violence can continue throughout the lifespan into senior years. For providers to understand the importance of screening for sexual violence, one must have a deep understanding of the prevalence, risk factors, and appropriate screening tools. Risk factors for victims of elder abuse include cognitive impairment, physical frailty, depression, and anxiety. Because these individuals may be cognitively impaired and are often socially isolated, they may make poor judgment in who they allow to care for them [23].

Limitations in surveys and the large amount of underreporting of sexual violence across the lifespan make the true incidence difficult to estimate. Estimates of elder abuse and sexual violence incidence vary, but it is clear that it is a significant public health problem. One study found that as many as 1 in 10 older adults have experienced elder abuse and it is estimated that more than 65% of elder abuse victims are women [24]. Another study in 2015 evaluating elder abuse in North and South America identified that prevalence was as high as 47% in adults with dementia, and 10% in the elderly who are cognitively intact [22]. The incidence of elder abuse varies widely ranging from 2% to 60%, and specific estimates for sexual violence are not available because of the significant differences in screening tools, definitions, and patient populations. However, 1 study did estimate that the prevalence of sexual mistreatment after reaching the age of 60 years was about 0.3% [25].

Screening for elder abuse, including sexual violence, has been encouraged since 1992 when the American Medical Association recommended providers in any practice setting should screen the geriatric population for signs of abuse. It was recommended that geriatric patients should be asked specifically about physical and emotional abuse and should be screened alone to avoid intimidation by potential abusers [22]. Because of the high prevalence of sexual violence and IPV, it is particularly important to screen patients who present with injuries or conditions that are suggestive of sexual violence.

Numerous governing bodies give recommendations on who should be screened and the frequency of screening. Much of the debate surrounding screening for sexual violence among elders involves a lack of evidence that screening improves health outcomes as well as the potential harms of screening [9]. The US Preventative Services Task Force guidelines currently state that there is insufficient evidence to recommend for or against sexual violence screening in older or vulnerable adults [18]. However, an ACOG committee statement supports the screening of patients older than 60 years for elder abuse and sexual violence to provide victims with the necessary medical and psychosocial resources [24]. In addition, the American Medical Association Code of Medical Ethics Opinion 8.10 recommends regular screening for physical, sexual, and psychological abuse [26]. Finally, the Health Resources and Services Administration Women's Preventive Services Guidelines support screening women for interpersonal and domestic violence annually and providing referrals for necessary services when abuse is identified [27].

Data suggest that providers are not currently screening for sexual violence regularly in practice. Initially, recommendations for screening in the geriatric population were not widely adopted because of the lack of efficient and validated screening tools, potential harms, including retaliation or abandonment by perpetrators, self-blame, and stigma associated with potentially positive screening results [28]. Two screening tools for elder abuse that are easily implemented and widely accepted into practice are the Brief Abuse Screen for the Elderly (BASE) and the Elder Assessment Instrument (EAI). The BASE takes about 1 minute to administer and allows the health care provider to identify suspected abuse and determine timing of intervention. The EAI tool has been used since the 1980s and includes 41 questions evaluating independence, medical and physical conditions, and social circumstances of the elderly patient to assess for elder abuse [22].

In addition, there are numerous screening tools specific to sexual and IPV that can be implemented into practice that have been discussed previously.

Table 1
Sexual violence screening tools

Tool	Length or estimated completion time	Targeted group
Abuse Assessment Screen	3 questions	Pregnant women
Brief Abuse Screen for the Elderly (BASE)	29 questions	Seniors & caregivers
Elder Assessment Instrument (EAI)	41 questions	Seniors
Humiliation, Afraid, Rape, Kick (HARK)	4 questions	Childbearing and seniors
Hurt, Insult, Threaten, Scream (HITS)	4 questions	Childbearing and seniors
Extended-Hurt, Insult, Threaten, Scream (E-HITS)	5 questions	Childbearing and seniors
Home, Education/Employment, Activities, Drugs, Sexuality, and Suicide/Depression (H.E.A.D.S.S.)	115 questions	High school & college age
Partner Violence Screen (PVS)	3 questions	Childbearing and seniors
SAFE Questionnaire	4 questions	All ages
STaT	3 questions	Childbearing and seniors
Woman Abuse Screening Tool (WAST)	8 questions	Childbearing

Additional tools include the SAFE questionnaire and the Abuse Assessment Screen. The SAFE questionnaire uses 4 questions that assess stress/safety, whether the patient is afraid/abused, if friends/family are aware of the abuse, and if they have an emergency plan. The Abuse Assessment Screen is a 3-item tool that assesses physical or sexual abuse within the last year and any abuse during pregnancy. Each of these tools have high sensitivity and specificity for identifying IPV. There are no nationally recognized guidelines for a "gold standard" screening tool when assessing sexual violence in the elderly. However, all organizations supporting screening for sexual violence do encourage providers to normalize inquiries about sexual violence and frame screening in a nonjudgmental manner to allow the patient to form a trusting and open relationship with their provider [22].

SUMMARY

Sexual violence has been identified as a serious public health issue affecting millions of women. Screening is a foundational step to intervention. Numerous tools are available for use in screening. Table 1 summarizes the various tools along with their length or estimated time for completion and targeted groups for use. Health care providers should be aware of sexual violence screening recommendations and use appropriate assessment tools with all women from adolescent through childbearing and senior years.

Disclosure

The authors disclose no conflicts of interest.

References

[1] Scope of the problem: Statistics. Rape, Abuse & Incest National Network. Available at: https://www.rainn.org/statistics/scope-problem. Accessed April 16, 2019.

[2] Preventing Intimate Partner Violence. Available at: https://www.cdc.gov/violencepreven-tion/. Accessed March 28, 2019.

[3] Dating matters: strategies to promote healthy teen relationships. Available at: https://www.cdc.gov/violenceprevention/datingmatters/science.html. Accessed March 28, 2019.

[4] Crawford-Jakubiak JE, Alderman EM, Leventhal JM. AAP Committee on Child Abuse and Neglect, AAP Committee on Adolescence. Care of the Adolescent After an Acute Sexual Assault. Pediatrics 2017;139(3):e20164243.

[5] Date rape: identification and management. Available at: https://www.uptodate.com. Accessed March 28, 2019.

[6] Reproductive and sexual coercion. Committee Opinion No. 554. American College of Obstetricians and Gynecologists. Obstet Gynecol 2013;121:411–5.

[7] David AK, Goldenrin JM, Adelman WP. HEEADSSS 3.0: the psychosocial interview for adolescents updated for a new century fueled by media. Contemp Pediatr 2014;January: 27–8.

[8] Women's Health Stats & Facts 2011. The American Congress of Obstetricians and Gynecologists. Available at: https://www.acog.org/-/media/NewsRoom/MediaKit.pdf. Accessed April 7, 2019.

[9] Weil A. Intimate partner violence: diagnosis and screening. In: Elmore JG, Kunins L, editors. UpToDate. 2019. Available at: www.uptodate.com 2019. Accessed April 7, 2019.

[10] Intimate Partner Violence. The Association of Women's Health, Obstetric, and Neonatal Nurses Position Statement. Available at: https://onlinelibrary.wiley.com/doi/epdf/10.1111/1552-6909.12567. Accessed April 7, 2019.

[11] Center for Disease Control and Prevention. Violence Prevention. In: National intimate partner and sexual violence survey: 2015 data Brief. Available at: https://www.cdc.gov/violenceprevention/pdf/2015data-brief508.pdf. Accessed April 7, 2019.

[12] Ford J, Soto-Marquez JG. Sexual assault victimization among straight, gay/lesbian, and bisexual college students. Violence Gend 2016;3(2):107–15.

[13] Wadsworth P, Degesie K, Kothari C, et al. Intimate partner violence during the perinatal period. J Nurse Pract 2018;14(10):753–8.

[14] Hahn CK, Gilmore AK, Orengo Aguayo R, et al. Perinatal intimate partner violence. Obstet Gynecol Clin North Am 2018;45(3):535–47.

[15] Chisholm CA, Bullock L, Ferguson JE II. Intimate partner violence and pregnancy: epidemiology and impact. Am J Obstet Gynecol 2017;217(2):141–4.

[16] The American Congress of Obstetricians and Gynecologists. Committee Opinion No. 518: intimate partner violence. Obstet Gynecol 2012;119(2):412–7.

[17] World Health Organization. Responding to intimate partner violence and sexual violence against women: WHO clinical and clinical guidelines. Geneva: World Health Organization; 2013. Available at: https://apps.who.int/iris/bitstream/handle/10665/85240/9789241548595_eng.pdf;jsessionid=948064763585E428CD1177F3190F7002?sequence=1. Accessed April 7, 2019.

[18] Sexual Assault. Committee Opinion No. 777. American Congress of Obstetricians and Gynecologists. Available at: https://www.acog.org/Clinical-Guidance-and-Publications/Committee-Opinions/Committee-on-Health-Care-for-Underserved-Women/Sexual-Assault?IsMobileSet=false. Accessed April 7, 2019.

[19] Final Recommendation Statement: intimate partner violence, elder abuse, and abuse of vulnerable adults: screening. U.S. Preventive Services Task Force. Available at: https://www.uspreventiveservicestaskforce.org/Page/Document/RecommendationStatementFinal/intimate-partner-violence-and-abuse-of-elderly-and-vulnerable-adults-screening1. Accessed April 7, 2019.

[20] Sohal H, Eldridge S, Feder G. The sensitivity and specificity of four questions (HARK) to identify intimate partner violence: a diagnostic accuracy study in general practice. BMC Fam Pract 2007;8:49.

[21] Basile KC, Hertz MF, Back SE. Intimate partner violence and sexual violence victimization assessment instruments for use in healthcare settings: version 1. Atlanta (GA): Centers for Disease Control and Prevention, National Center for Injury Prevention and Control; 2007. https://www.cdc.gov/violenceprevention/pdf/ipv/ipvandsvscreening.pdf. Accessed May 7, 2019.

[22] Halphen JM, Dyer CB. Elder mistreatment: abuse, neglect, and financial exploitation. In: Post TW, editor. UpToDate. 2019. Available at: www.uptodate.com 2019. Accessed April 6, 2019.

[23] Dong XQ. Elder abuse: systematic review and implications for practice. J Am Geriatr Soc 2015;63(6):1214–38.

[24] The American Congress of Obstetricians and Gynecologists. Committee Opinion No. 568: elder abuse and women's health. Obstet Gynecol 2013;122:187–91.

[25] Acierno R, Hernandez MA, Amstadter AB, et al. Prevalence and correlates of emotional, physical, sexual, and financial abuse and potential neglect in the United States: the national elder mistreatment study. Am J Public Health 2010;100:292–7.

[26] Preventing, identifying & treating violence & abuse: code of medical ethics opinion 8.10. American Medical Association. Available at: https://www.ama-assn.org/delivering-care/ethics/preventing-identifying-treating-violence-abuse. Accessed April 7, 2019.

[27] Women's Preventive Services Guidelines. Health Resources & Services Administration. Available at: https://www.hrsa.gov/womens-guidelines-2016/index.html. Accessed April 9, 2019.

[28] Fulmer T, Guadagno L, Bitondo Dyer C, et al. Progress in elder abuse screening and assessment instruments. J Am Geriatr Soc 2004;52(2):297.

Advances in Family Practice Nursing 2 (2020) 87–102

ADVANCES IN FAMILY PRACTICE NURSING

Wellness and Disease Self-Management Mobile Health Apps Evaluated by the Mobile Application Rating Scale

Melissa Stec, DNP, CNM, APRN, FACNM, FAAN[a],*,
Megan W. Arbour, PhD, CNM, CNE, FACNM[b]

[a]SUNY Downstate Health Sciences University, 450 Clarkson Ave MS 22 Brooklyn, NY 11203, USA; [b]Frontier Nursing University, 195 School St Hyden, KY 41749, USA

Keywords
- Telemedicine • Mobile applications • Smartphone • Chronic disease
- Self-management

Key points

- Accurate health information can empower patients to take charge of their own disease management.
- Mobile health apps can provide accurate information and encourage disease self-management.
- Use of the Mobile Application Rating Scale (MARS) tool can assist providers in choosing highly effective apps for patients.

INTRODUCTION

As the US population of baby boomers ages, 90% of the nation's 3.3 trillion health care dollars are spent on the management of mental health and chronic disease [1]. Primary care providers often experience time constraints that decrease their ability to optimally manage chronic illnesses and provide comprehensive patient education [2]. As a result, clinicians are increasingly in search of opportunities for patients to use illness or disease self-management tools to help alleviate the burden of chronic disease. Self-management of disease plays an important role in disease progression and

*Corresponding author. E-mail address: melissa.stec@downstate.edu

https://doi.org/10.1016/j.yfpn.2020.01.003
2589-420X/20/© 2020 Elsevier Inc. All rights reserved.

prognosis because patients take ownership and responsibility for their health and wellness.

Accurate health information can empower patients to take charge of their own disease management and play a key role in their care [3]. Mobile technology has now reached a tipping point with more devices, such as smartphones and tablets, in use than traditional computers [4]. These mobile technologies can be a catalyst for disease self-management, allowing patients to play a key role in their health care. Research shows that programs focused on disease self-management can be tailored to specific populations and use a diverse set of strategies that have been shown to improve outcomes [5]. Mobile apps are a convenient, accessible option for disease or illness self-management that integrate evidence-based interventions such as feedback, interaction, and patient support [6]. These apps can support self-management by using modalities that provide evidence-based information and educational resources as well as encouraging medication compliance and symptom monitoring [7,8].

BACKGROUND/LITERATURE
Behavior change
Changes in behavior are often required for health improvement. Some health changes are recommended at a population level, with policy and guideline recommendations, such as dietary guidelines to reduce heart disease. Often, these changes do not work as successfully as hoped because the change-makers act in reaction to the need for change rather than fixing the instigating problem [9]. In the example given earlier, specific components of the diet may not be as much to blame as overeating or lack of activity in cardiovascular morbidity. The same may be true for individuals seeking to make health changes. The instigating behavior needs to be addressed before successful and positive change can be made. Changes in behavior are not easy to make, and require significant planning and thought [9]. Mobile health (mHealth) apps that are evidence based have the opportunity to be the well-thought-out change-making impetus. The US Food and Drug Administration recognizes the utility of digital health tools, including apps and clinical decision support software, for health improvement [10].

Once the instigating behavior is identified and behavioral changes have been initiated, maintenance of the changed behavior is often tricky and requires attention to the motives for change, resources and habits related to the change, as well as influences in the individual's life [11]. One way to manage this is through the use of disease or illness self-management apps. Zhao and colleagues [12] and others note that positive health behavior change can occur and be maintained as a result of app usage. Characteristics of apps that led to retained behavior change compared with apps that did not retain behavior changes include less time consumption, user-friendly design, real-time feedback, individualized elements of the app, detailed information, and health professional involvement [12].

Smartphone usage

Smartphone usage seems ubiquitous, and some people assume that mHealth apps are also used by most individuals. Clinicians often use mHealth apps to access up-to-date clinical information [8], and some patients use apps to improve their health and wellness [13]. Krebs and Duncan [14] conducted a cross-sectional survey of more than 1600 mobile phone users in the United States. They determined that roughly half had downloaded a health-related mobile app, but approximately half of those had stopped using the app because of time factors, costs, and loss of interest. This finding indicates that there is a perfect combination of factors in place for which clinicians can recommend apps: (1) clinicians are very busy and seek to empower their patients to use self-management apps for chronic disease management; (2) patients have and use mobile devices; (3) clinicians know the characteristics of apps that help patients maintain their behavior changes [12]. How do clinicians know which apps to recommend?

When clinicians choose to recommend an app for patient health care improvement, it is helpful to know the quality of the app and whether it will be one that leads to retained behavior change [13]. Clinicians may also consider whether the app has associated costs of time or money, and whether the benefit of usage outweighs these costs. The Mobile Application Rating Scale (MARS) is designed to evaluate mHealth apps based on 5 key quality areas: engagement, functionality, aesthetics, information, and subjective quality [15]. Each of these main quality scoring criteria are further divided into subscales (Table 1). Each of the 5 subscales is averaged for a maximum mean score of 5, with 5 indicating highest quality and 0 indicating lowest quality for each subscale. Use of the MARS tool provides quantitative data for ranking mobile apps that can be used to assist clinicians in choosing appropriate technologies for management of illness.

Numerous researchers have evaluated mHealth apps using the MARS tool and have published the detailed reports. Recommended apps may exist on the iOS platform, the Android platform, or both, in which case they are called agnostic or device agnostic. This article highlights the highest-rated mHealth apps for areas of adult chronic disease management, as well as selecting primary care topics for adolescents and older adults, as reported using the MARS tool.

ADULTS/CHRONIC DISEASE MANAGEMENT

Hypertension

Globally, 1 in 5 people have a diagnosis of hypertension [16]. Although hypertension requires careful monitoring and management, it also carries with it a risk of stroke and kidney disease. Mobile apps for management of hypertension should reflect national evidence-based guidelines for the management of hypertension but should also include 5 key features: the ability to export data, send reminders, analyze data, record time, and provide education [17]. These features allow several aspects of self-management as well collaborative

Table 1
Modified Mobile Application Rating Scale scoring criteria

Criteria	Subscales	Subscale description
Engagement	Entertainment	Is the app entertaining?
	Interest	Is the app interesting to use?
	Customization	Does the app retain settings?
	Interactivity	Does the app allow input or provide feedback?
	Target group	Is the app appropriate for the target audience?
Functionality	Performance	How accurately do the app features work?
	Ease of use	How easy is it to learn to use the app?
	Navigation	Is moving between screens logical?
	Gestural design	Are interactions consistent and intuitive?
Aesthetics	Layout	Is arrangement and size appropriate?
	Graphics	Are the graphics and resolution high quality?
	Visual appeal	How does the app look?
Information	Accuracy	Is the description accurate?
	Goals	Does the app have specific goals?
	Quality	Is the information relevant and correct?
	Quantity	IS the information comprehensive?
	Visual information	Is the visual explanation of concepts correct?
	Credibility	Does the app come from a legitimate source?
	Evidence based	Is the app verified by evidence?

Data from Stoyanov SR, Hides L, Kavanagh DJ, et al. Mobile app rating scale: A new tool for assessing the quality of health mobile apps. JMIR Mhealth Uhealth. 2015;3(1):e27. https://doi.org/10.2196/mhealth.3422 [doi].

management with a health care provider. In a study regarding hypertension apps, Jamaladin and colleagues [17] screened 4613 apps. Of those, 184 met inclusion criteria (104 Android, 80 iOS) and each was then evaluated using the MARS criteria. The top 2 apps available in English were AMICOMED BP (MARS 3.7, iOS) and Beurer HealthManager (3.7, Android). One additional app, Bloeddruk (MARS 4.1, Android) was rated higher but is only available in Dutch. AMICOMED was the only app that included all of the identified key features. Clinicians may choose to recommend this app to patients who seek to play an active role in their hypertension management.

Chronic kidney disease

When discussing hypertension, providers often must consider comorbidities, including chronic kidney disease (CKD). These diagnoses require dietary and other lifestyle modifications and symptom tracking that can be managed using mobile technologies. Most importantly, patients need high-quality information to accurately manage their conditions [18]. Managing a renal diet can be a challenge for patients who are also managing multiple medications. Lambert and colleagues [18] reviewed mobile applications to assist patients in dietary management, and 1066 apps were identified using specific keywords. Of these, 21 apps were eligible for full review and 10 were considered accurate and evidence based. Although no specific app scored well in all domains, 2 apps were highlighted in the recommendations. MyFood Coach (MARS = 3.8, agnostic) and H20 Overload (MARS = 3.7, agnostic) scored well in terms of information quality and technical functionality.

Siddique and colleagues [19] reviewed apps useful for nutrition tracking and medication compliance for patients with CKD. They screened 431 apps for specific keywords, and 196 met inclusion criteria. After secondary screening for functionality and features, 12 apps were scored using the MARS tool. My Kidneys, My Health Handbook (MARS = 4.68, agnostic), and My Food Coach (MARS = 4.48, agnostic) were the two highest-rated MARS apps in this study [19]. The investigators recognized that a more comprehensive app for patients with chronic renal disease should be developed that incorporate techniques such as feedback and caregiver interaction [18,19].

Heart failure and self-care management

Heart failure affects at least 26 million people worldwide and is responsible for $31 billion in health care expenditures [20]. Heart failure–related exacerbations are the most common reason for hospitalization in older adults [21]. Avoiding admission to the hospital is a primary goal for providers and is not possible without patient self-management components such as daily weight monitoring, fluid restriction, dietary modifications, and exercise. Masterson Creber and colleagues [21] reviewed targeted apps, considering supporting symptoms and self-care management in relation to these areas. In all, 3636 apps were searched and 164 chosen for further evaluation. After secondary screening, 34 met the inclusion criteria. Apps were additionally screened for 8 specific self-care behaviors recommended by the Heart Failure Society of America. Two apps, Heart Failure Health Storylines (MARS = 4.6, agnostic) and Symple (MARS = 4.1, iOS), were evaluated to have the most options for symptom tracking. In addition, Heart Failure Health Storylines also included all of the Heart Failure Society of America behaviors. Further work is needed to develop an app inclusive of evidence-based guidelines for symptom monitoring and self-care.

Woods and colleagues [22] conducted mixed-methods research examining consumer mobile app use for the self-management of heart failure. Although the sample size was small (n = 6 enrolled patients), the investigators concluded that integration of mobile technology was difficult because of the well-established self-care and self-management techniques being used by patients. Essentially, patients with heart failure already had a set self-care and self-management routine, and did not see the need or desire to integrate mobile technology into this routine. As a subtheme of the study, participants rated Care4myHeart (MARS = 3.53, agnostic), an mHealth app that was developed within their health care organization [22].

Smoking cessation

In the United States, 34.3 million adults are smokers [23]. Smoking and tobacco use is the largest preventable cause of death and disease in the United States, with smoking-related illnesses costing $300 billion a year (Centers for Disease Control and Prevention). There is evidence to support behavioral interventions for smoking cessation, such as motivation, advice, counseling, and pharmacologic support [24]. Thornton and colleagues [25] conducted a review of free app-based smoking cessation tools in an effort to overcome barriers to cessation, such as lack of resources and lack of clinician knowledge or time. The review initially yielded 2644 apps and, of those, 651 met initial criteria. On secondary review, 112 apps were reviewed in full, yielding 6 high-quality apps. My QuitBuddy (MARS = 4.9, agnostic) and quitSTART (MARS = 4.6, agnostic) had the highest mean MARS scores and subjective quality scores. Each app focuses on education, monitoring, goal settings, and advice that can assist smokers in their goal toward smoking cessation [25].

Mental health

Nearly 1 in 5 adults in the United States live with a mental illness inclusive of many conditions that are moderate to severe [26]. In addition, 17.3 million adults have had at least 1 depressive episode [27]. Increasing evidence is available showing that mobile apps are effective in the management of a variety of mental health disorders, including anxiety, depression, and bipolar disorder [28]. Neary and Schueller [28] summarized data based on the PsyberGuide (https://psyberguide.org/) Web platform. PsyberGuide is a not-for-profit initiative that maintains an online consumer guide for digital mental health products. This Web platform provides available evidence and relevant information on each of numerous mental health and wellness apps. PsyberGuide uses the MARS tool to evaluate these apps and classifies this as an user experience score. Neary and Schueller [28] reported that 7 mental health–related apps have MARS scores more than 4.5. Stop, Breathe, & Think (MARS = 4.75, agnostic), Headspace (MARS = 4.74, agnostic), and Buddhify (MARS = 4.51, agnostic) are specific to self-management techniques such as meditation and mindfulness. Peak (MARS 4.52, agnostic) and Pacifica (MARS = 4.7, agnostic) are two highly rated apps that focus on cognitive behavior therapy skills [28]. Providers can access the PsyberGuide Web site to differentiate effective highly rated apps by diagnosis or by self-management technique, to further individualize treatment recommendations.

Sleep management

Adults need 7 or more hours of sleep per night for the best health [29,30]. Adults who routinely get less than 7 hours of sleep are more likely to report a variety of chronic conditions such as heart disease, arthritis, depression, and diabetes [29]. Adolescents need an increased number of hours of sleep, requiring 8 to 10 hours per night. Mobile apps that incorporate sleep management interventions have the potential to improve health care outcomes for patients with sleep deficiencies [31]. Choi and colleagues [31] identified 2431 apps based on keyword searches related to sleep and sleep management. After screening and assessment by description, 148 apps were downloaded. After further review, 73 apps were reviewed using the MARS tool and the Institute for Healthcare Informatics app functionality score (IMS). Four apps were high performing, including Sleep Center Free (MARS = 4.0, iOS), Good Morning

Alarm Clock (MARS = 3.7, agnostic), Sleep as Android Unlock (MARS = 4.0, Android), and Samsung Health (MARS = 3.7, Android). Of these, 3 of the 4 (Good Morning Alarm Clock, Sleep as Android Unlock, Samsung Health) include 11 IMS criteria, including app capabilities such as inform, instruct, record, collect data, and communicate.

Pain

Chronic pain is an epidemic in the United States, with an estimated 20.4% of American adults experiencing chronic pain annually [32]. Pain is a major indicator as to why patients seek treatment. The overprescribing of narcotic pain medication has led providers to seek alternative methods for the management of chronic pain [33]. Salazar and colleagues [34] reviewed mobile apps for the management of pain using the MARS tool. Forty-seven apps were identified using keyword search and, after screening, 18 apps were included in the review. Three apps scored more than 4.0 using the MARS tool, Pain Companion (MARS = 4.35, Android), Manage My Pain (MARS = 4.22, Android), and My Pain Diary (MARS = 4.02, iOS). Pain Companion has the most focus points, including increase happiness/well-being, goal setting, entertainment, relationships, and physical health. Several apps are available depending on the individual app functionality needs of the patient, and also include alternative resources for patients with chronic pain [34].

ADOLESCENTS

Targeting the adolescent population for app usage for the self-management of disease or illness is challenging because of their developmental stages that are different than those of adults. In addition, many app manufacturers do not include adolescents in app development or do not test their efficacy with adolescents [35,36].

Diet, physical activity, and sedentary behavior

Interventions promoting healthy behaviors and physical activity are widely sought after for adolescent populations. Schoeppe and colleagues [37] reviewed mobile apps to determine the content and quality of apps regarding diet, physical activity, and sedentary behavior. Apps were evaluated using the MARS tool and the behavior change techniques (BCTs) interventions available in the app. Initially based on keyword searches, 42,595 apps were identified on these topics and 132 apps were screen based on descriptions. In all, 25 apps were selected for full screening based on inclusion criteria. GoNoodle Kids (MARS = 4.4, BCT = 8, agnostic) and Fitbit (MARS = 4.3, BCT = 8, agnostic) provided both excellent MARS scores and an acceptable number of BCTs [37]. Providers can select appropriate apps for adolescents based on specific goals for promotion of health or treatment of disease.

Asthma

According to the World Health Organization, 235 million people worldwide have a diagnosis of asthma [38]. Asthma is a chronic airway disease characterized by respiratory symptoms and is the most common chronic disease among children. Effective disease self-management of asthma can reduce the burden for both patients and providers, and mobile-based technology can provide a low-cost and effective intervention [39,40]. Mobile apps work to improve self-management by providing medication reminders and symptom tracking while facilitating patient-provider communication [7].

The aim of Tinschert and colleagues [39] was to identify apps useful in asthma self-management. These apps are not specific to adolescents but may be useful for them. Based on screening, 523 apps were identified and, of these, 46 were downloaded and an additional 8 were duplicates. Thirty-eight apps were fully screened with Wizdy Pets (MARS 4.55, agnostic) and Asthma Health (MARS $\frac{1}{4}$ 4.45, iOS) scoring highest in the study. High-scoring apps in the study included multiple available functions, BCTs, and gamification components. Ramsey and colleagues [7] also screened available apps for asthma for the presence of BCTs, initially identifying 95 apps. Of these apps identified by BCTs, 40 apps remained after screening and 23 were fully reviewed once duplicates were removed. Most apps evaluated included a mean of 4 BCTs such as instruction, behavior-health link, self-monitoring, feedback, teach to use prompts/cues, and consequences. Three apps, AsthmaMD (MARS = 4.23, agnostic), Kiss myAsthma (MARS = 4.22, agnostic), and My Breathefree (MARS = 3.79, agnostic), included at least 8 BCTs, with AsthmaMD scoring the highest on the MARS scale. Of the 2 studies, 1 app, Asthma Health (MARS = 4.45 and 4.5, iOS, 5 BCTs), was well ranked on the MARS scale and contained an adequate number of BCTs [7,39].

OLDER ADULTS
Balance and falls
Falls are the second leading cause of unintentional injury deaths worldwide [41]. Approximately 37 million people experience a fall requiring medical attention annually, with adults aged 65 years and older comprising the largest number of fatal falls [41]. These statistics provide evidence that balance is an important aspect of care for older adults. In a 2018 study, Reyes and colleagues [42] examined apps targeted to improve or maintain balance. Specific search criteria were not included in the report; however, 5 apps were included for full evaluation and scoring. UStabalize was the highest-rated app (MARS = 4, iOS), but the only app specifically for older adults was Senior Balance quiz (MARS = 3.4, iOS). These apps are intended to help give information and train the users to obtain better balance [42]. Note that all balance-related apps are only available for iOS.

Arthritis
Arthritis is a chronic inflammatory disease affecting 55 million people nationwide [43]. Symptom management is an integral part of treatment of arthritis, and mobile technologies can assist patients in tracking and monitoring their symptoms. Grainger and colleagues [44] conducted a review of available

Table 2
Apps by category and Mobile Application Rating Scale score

Age group	App topic	App name	MARS score	Platform	Features	Reference
Adults	Hypertension	AMICOMED BP	3.7	iOS	• Sync with clinician • Track blood pressures • View history	Jamaladin et al [17], 2018
		Beurer HealthManager	3.7	Android	• See blood pressure trends • Tracks weight, blood pressure, blood glucose, activity, sleep, and pulse oximetry	
	CKD	H2O Overload	3.7	iOS	• Easy to switch between screens Tracks fluid consumption, weight, and blood pressure • Provides alert as to when to notify doctor	Lambert et al [18], 2017
		My Kidneys, My Health Handbook	4.68	Agnostic	• Provides education about disease and how to explain to family and friends • Encourages lifestyle changes	Jamaladin et al [17], 2018
		My Food Coach	4.48	Agnostic	• Provides recipes and nutritional information for individuals with kidney disease • User-friendly design	
	Heart failure	Heart Failure Health Storylines	4.6	Agnostic	• Can track vital signs, symptoms, weight, medications, journal feelings, and moods • Note appointments	Masterson Creber et al [21], 2016
		Symple Symptom Tracker	4.1	iOS	• Keep track of all health components in 1 place • Symptoms, step count, sleep statistics, heart rate, and so forth • Take photos of meds or meals • List questions in a journal • Track and note trends	

(continued on next page)

Table 2
(continued)

Age group	App topic	App name	MARS score	Platform	Features	Reference
	Smoking cessation	Care4myHeart	3.53	Agnostic	• Create a PDF file to bring to clinician	Woods et al [22], 2019
		Quite Now: My QuitBuddy	4.9	Agnostic	• Not commercially available • Set Personal goals • Track Progress • See how much money has been saved • Alerts keep patient on track • Social interaction with others who are trying to quit	Thornton et al [25], 2017
		quitSTART - Quit Smoking	4.6	Agnostic	• Earn badges for smoke-free milestones • Identify triggers • Helps to manage cravings • Calculates time away from smoking • Tracks moods • Provides distractions and alerts • Social media component	
	Mental health/ CBT	Peak	4.52	Agnostic	• Brain training, improves cognitive skills • User friendly • Well designed	Neary & Schueller [28], 2018
		Pacifica	4.7	Agnostic	• Helps with stress and anxiety through guided meditation, self-care, on-demand help • Mood trackers	
	Sleep management	Good Morning Alarm Clock	3.7	Agnostic	• Sleep timer and tracker that uses phone microphone • Includes sound machine, tracks sleep cycles	Choi et al [31], 2018
		Sleep as Android Unlock	4.0	Android	• Alarm clock, sleep cycle tracker	
		Samsung Health	3.7	Android	• Track numerous health components in 1 place (dietary intake, physical activity, water, caffeine, heart rate, blood pressure, weight, and so forth)	

				Features	Platform	Reference
Adoles-cents	Pain	Pain Companion	4.35	• Tracks sleep cycles • Records pain levels and provides graphs • Tracks fatigue, mood • Has messaging feature • Contains educational information on pain management	Android	Salazar et al [34], 2018
		My Pain Diary	4.02	• Provides trackers for multiple chronic diagnoses • Maps pain location • Records pain calendar • Contains medication log	iOS	
	Diet, physical activity, and sedentary behavior	GoNoodle Kids	4.4	• Several modalities to get children on the move • New content weekly	Agnostic	Schoeppe et al [37], 2017
		FitBit	4.3	• Caters to multiple age groups • Goal-setting feature • Tracks steps and calories • Includes family group	Agnostic	
	Asthma management	Wizdy Pets	4.55	• Uses gamification for children to manage asthma • Allows children to collect badges • Helps children learn asthma management techniques	Agnostic	Tinschert et al [39], 2017
		AsthmaHealth	4.45	• Contains medication reminders • Tracks symptoms • Reviews trends • Gives feedback	iOS	
		AsthmaMD	4.23	• Charts severity based on peak flow measurements • Interacts with providers • Has medication function	Agnostic	Ramsey et al [7], 2019.
		Kiss myAsthma	4.22	• Accesses emergency help • Uses medication reminders • Has educational component	Agnostic	
		My Breathefree	3.79	• Uses peak flow measurements to track symptoms • Medication reminders	Agnostic	

(continued on next page)

Table 2
(continued)

Age group	App topic	App name	MARS score	Platform	Features	Reference
Older adults	Balance and falls	UStabalize	4.0	iOS	• Provides interaction with providers • Uses gamification to help improve balance • Allows users to take balance challenges	Reyes et al, [42] 2018
		Senior Balance quiz	3.4	iOS	• Provides quiz to help seniors make life changes to avoid falls	
	Arthritis	RheumaHelper	4.26	Agnostic	• Toolbox of disease activity • Best for providers • Evidence-based material	Grainger et al [44], 2017
		Arthritis Power	3.41	Agnostic	• Track symptoms and well-being • Medication tracking • Shares information with providers	

Abbreviation: CBT, cognitive behavior therapy.

apps for education and symptom tracking regarding arthritis. Using keyword searches, 937 apps (iOS and Android) were identified. After screening, 19 apps were included in the review. The review included scoring using the MARS tool and screening for adherence with monitoring recommendations from the American College of Rheumatology (ACR) and the European League Against Rheumatism (EULAR). On review, there were no apps that scored greater than 4.0 on the MARS and included all ACR and EULAR instruments; however, 6 apps scored more than 4.0 using the MARS tool [44]. Rheuma-Helper (MARS = 4.26, agnostic) included disease activity scores but lacked a data-tracking tool. Arthritis Power (MARS = 3.41, agnostic) included ACR and EULAR–recommended composite disease activity score [44]. Clinicians need to weigh the benefit of having a higher MARS-ranked app (Rheuma-Helper) with one that includes national clinical guidelines (Arthritis Power).

IMPLICATIONS FOR PRACTICE

Self-management of disease and health promotion through the use of mobile apps is an area of rapid growth, and the use of mobile devices is proliferative [42]. Clinicians have the opportunity to empower patients to take charge of their wellness and improve their disease self-management through the use of mobile apps. Mobile apps have a variety of functional components, including the ability to transmit data to clinicians, incorporate the latest clinical practice guidelines, provide patient feedback, use BCTs, and be customizable to individual patients. The topics reviewed here are commonly encountered primary care topics for adults, older adults, and adolescents, and the best apps for each topic are highlighted in Table 2. The MARS is a valid and reliable tool that has been tested in a variety of health topics and thousands of apps [15]. Apps with highly rated MARS scores can be trusted for recommendation by clinicians.

Incorporation of apps into clinical practice for clinician usage, or for recommendation to patients, can seem overwhelming. Clinicians are encouraged to choose a single app to try, and determine how best to incorporate it or find a specific patient who might be a good initial user. If it does not work well, it is appropriate for the clinician to try again with another app or another patient. This process helps clinicians' confidence in app usage and in giving recommendations [8].

References

[1] Centers for Disease Control and Prevention. National center for chronic disease prevention and health promotion (NCCDPHP): health and economic costs of chronic disease. 2019. Available at: https://www.cdc.gov/chronicdisease/about/costs/index.htm#ref1. Accessed September 18, 2019.

[2] Dugdale DC, Epstein R, Pantilat SZ. Time and the patient-physician relationship. J Gen Intern Med 1999;14(S1):S34–40.

[3] Coulter A, Parsons S, Askham J. Policy brief: where are the patients in decision-making about their own care?. 2008. Available at: https://www.who.int/management/general/decisionmaking/WhereArePatientsinDecisionMaking.pdf. Accessed August 15, 2019.

[4] Statcounter. Share of mobile device owners worldwide from 2011 to 2016, by number of devices owned. 2016. Available at: http://gs.statcounter.com/press/mobile-and-tablet-internet-usage-exceeds-desktop-for-first-time-worldwide. Accessed September 12, 2019.

[5] Grady PA, Gough LL. Self-management: a comprehensive approach to management of chronic conditions. Rev Panam Salud Publica 2015;37(3):187–94.

[6] Brouwer W, Kroeze W, Crutzen R, et al. Which intervention characteristics are related to more exposure to internet-delivered healthy lifestyle promotion interventions? A systematic review. J Med Internet Res 2011;13(1):23–41.

[7] Ramsey RR, Caromody JK, Voorhees SE, et al. A systematic evaluation of asthma management apps examining behavior change techniques. J Allergy Clin Immunol Pract 2019;7(8): 2583–91.

[8] Arbour MW, Stec MA. Mobile applications for women's health and midwifery care: a pocket reference for the 21st century. J Midwifery Womens Health 2018;63(3):330–4.

[9] Kelly MP, Barker M. Why is changing health-related behaviour so difficult? Public Health 2016;136:109–16.

[10] U.S. Food & Drug Administration. Mobile medical applications. 2015. Available at: https://www.fda.gov/medicaldevices/digitalhealth/mobilemedicalapplications/default.htm. Accessed August 31, 2017.

[11] Kwasnicka D, Dombrowski SU, White M, et al. Theoretical explanations for maintenance of behaviour change: a systematic review of behaviour theories. Health Psychol Rev 2016;10(3):277–96.

[12] Zhao J, Freeman B, Li M. Can mobile phone apps influence people's health behavior change? an evidence review. J Med Internet Res 2016;18(11):e287.

[13] Stec MA, Arbour MW, Hines HF. Client-Centered mobile health care applications: using the mobile application rating scale instrument for Evidence-Based evaluation. J Midwifery Womens Health 2019;64(3):324–9.

[14] Krebs P, Duncan DT. Health app use among US mobile phone owners: a national survey. JMIR Mhealth Uhealth 2015;3(4):e101.

[15] Stoyanov SR, Hides L, Kavanagh DJ, et al. Mobile app rating scale: a new tool for assessing the quality of health mobile apps. JMIR Mhealth Uhealth 2015;3(1):e27.

[16] World Health Organization. Raised blood pressure (SBP ≥140 OR DBP ≥90), crude (%) data by WHO region. 2017. Available at: http://apps.who.int/gho/data/view.-main.NCDBPCREGv?lang=en. Accessed September 15, 2019.

[17] Jamaladin H, van de Belt TH, Luijpers LC, et al. Mobile apps for blood pressure monitoring: systematic search in app stores and content analysis. JMIR Mhealth Uhealth 2018;6(11): e187.

[18] Lambert K, Mullan J, Mansfield K, et al. Should we recommend renal Diet–Related apps to our patients? an evaluation of the quality and health literacy demand of renal Diet–Related mobile applications. J Ren Nutr 2017;27(6):430–8.

[19] Siddique AB, Krebs M, Alvarez S, et al. Mobile apps for the care management of chronic kidney and end-stage renal diseases: systematic search in app stores and evaluation. JMIR Mhealth Uhealth 2019;7(9):e12604.

[20] Savarese G, Lund LH, Department of Cardiology, Karolinska University Hospital, Stockholm, Sweden, Division of Cardiology, Department of Medicine, Karolinska Insitutet, Stockholm, Sweden. Global public health burden of heart failure. Card Fail Rev 2017;3(1): 7–11.

[21] Masterson Creber RM, Maurer MS, Reading M, et al. Review and analysis of existing mobile phone apps to support heart failure symptom monitoring and self-care management using the mobile application rating scale (MARS). JMIR Mhealth Uhealth 2016;4(2):e74.

[22] Woods LS, Duff J, Roehrer E, et al. Patients' experiences of using a consumer mHealth app for self-management of heart failure: mixed-methods study. JMIR Hum Factors 2019;6(2): e13009.

[23] Centers for Disease Control and Prevention (CDC). Smoking and tobacco use: fast facts and fact sheets. 2019. Available at: https://www.cdc.gov/tobacco/data_statistics/fact_-sheets/index.htm. Accessed September 18, 2019.

[24] Roberts NJ, Kerr SM, Smith SMS. Behavioral interventions associated with smoking cessation in the treatment of tobacco use. Health Serv Insights 2013;2013(6):79–85.

[25] Thornton L, Quinn C, Birrell L, et al. Free smoking cessation mobile apps available in australia: a quality review and content analysis. Aust N Z J Public Health 2017;41(6): 625–30.

[26] National Institute of Mental Health (NIMH). Mental illness. 2019. Available at: https:// www.nimh.nih.gov/health/statistics/mental-illness.shtml. Accessed September 18, 2019.

[27] National Institute of Mental Health (NIMH). Major depression. 2019. Available at: https:// www.nimh.nih.gov/health/statistics/major-depression.shtml. Accessed September 18, 2019.

[28] Neary M, Schueller SM. State of the field of mental health apps. Cogn Behav Pract 2018;25(4):531–7.

[29] Hirshkowitz M, Whiton K, Albert SM, et al. National sleep foundation's updated sleep duration recommendations. Sleep Health 2015;1(4):233–43.

[30] Consensus Conference Panel, Watson NF, Badr MS, et al. Joint consensus statement of the american academy of sleep medicine and sleep research society on the recommended amount of sleep for a healthy adult: methodology and discussion. J Clin Sleep Med 2015;11(8):931–52.

[31] Choi YK, Demiris G, Lin S, et al. Smartphone applications to support sleep self-management: review and evaluation. J Clin Sleep Med 2018;14(10):1783–90.

[32] Dahlhamer J, Lucas J, Zelaya C, et al. Prevalence of chronic pain and high-impact chronic pain among adults - united states, 2016. MMWR Morb Mortal Wkly Rep 2018;67(36): 1001–6.

[33] National Academies of Sciences, Engineering, and Medicine, Health and Medicine Division, Board on Health Sciences Policy, et al. Pain management and the opioid epidemic: balancing societal and individual benefits and risks of prescription opioid use. Washington, DC: National Academies Press; 2017.

[34] Salazar A, de Sola H, Failde I, et al. Measuring the quality of mobile apps for the management of pain: systematic search and evaluation using the mobile app rating scale. JMIR Mhealth Uhealth 2018;6(10):e10718.

[35] Majeed-Ariss R, Baildam E, Campbell M, et al. Apps and adolescents: a systematic review of adolescents' use of mobile phone and tablet apps that support personal management of their chronic or long-term physical conditions. J Med Internet Res 2015;17(12):e287.

[36] Dute DJ, Bemelmans WJE, Breda J. Using mobile apps to promote a healthy lifestyle among adolescents and students: a review of the theoretical basis and lessons learned. JMIR Mhealth Uhealth 2016;4(2):e39.

[37] Schoeppe S, Alley S, Rebar AL, et al. Apps to improve diet, physical activity and sedentary behaviour in children and adolescents: a review of quality, features and behaviour change techniques. Int J Behav Nutr Phys Act 2017;14(1):83.

[38] World Health Organization. Chronic respiratory diseases: asthma. 2019. Available at: https://www.who.int/respiratory/asthma/en/. Accessed September 18, 2019.

[39] Tinschert P, Jakob R, Barata F, et al. The potential of mobile apps for improving asthma self-management: a review of publicly available and well-adopted asthma apps. JMIR Mhealth Uhealth 2017;5(8):e113.

[40] Wu AC. The promise of improving asthma control using mobile health. J Allergy Clin Immunol Pract 2016;4(4):738–9.

[41] World Health Organization. Falls. 2019. Available at: https://www.who.int/en/news-room/fact-sheets/detail/falls. Accessed September 18, 2019.

[42] Reyes A, Qin P, Brown CA. A standardized review of smartphone applications to promote balance for older adults. Disabil Rehabil 2018;40(6):690–6.

[43] Centers for Disease Control and Prevention (CDC). Arthritis national statistics. 2018. Available at: https://www.cdc.gov/arthritis/data_statistics/national-statistics.html. Accessed September 18, 2019.

[44] Grainger R, Townsley H, White B, et al. Apps for people with rheumatoid arthritis to monitor their disease activity: a review of apps for best practice and quality. JMIR Mhealth Uhealth 2017;5(2):e7.

Advances in Family Practice Nursing 2 (2020) 103–113

ADVANCES IN FAMILY PRACTICE NURSING

Hypertensive Disorders in Pregnancy
Implications for Primary Care

Tonja M.A. Santos, CNM, MSN

Baystate Midwifery Education Program, Baystate Midwifery and Women's Health, 689 Chestnut Street, Springfield, MA 01199, USA

Keywords

- Hypertension • Preeclampsia • Racial disparities • Cardiovascular risk
- Lifestyle modification • Reproductive justice

Key points

- Cardiovascular disease is a major contributor to morbidity and mortality for women in the United States and worldwide.
- Rates of hypertensive disorders in pregnancy are increasing. At the same time, the risk factors associated with these hypertensive disorders are also on the increase.
- By recognizing women at risk for hypertensive disorders in pregnancy and working with them before, during, and after pregnancy we can reduce both pregnancy-related and lifetime risks.
- Mitigating these risk factors could also decrease racial disparities in maternal morbidity and mortality.

INTRODUCTION

With the growing burden of coronary heart disease (CHD) and cerebrovascular disease (CVD) on women worldwide, it is imperative that the medical community take every opportunity to understand contributing factors to eliminate or mitigate risk for women over their lifetime. Hypertensive disorders of pregnancy (HDP), the most common group of pregnancy-related complications [1], are the leading causes of maternal morbidity and mortality in the United States and worldwide [2,3]. As rates of obesity, comorbid chronic medical conditions, and pregnancies in women considered of "advanced maternal age" (≥35 years at time of delivery) continue to increase, so too will rates of HDP [4].

E-mail address: Tonja.santosCNM@baystatehealth.org

https://doi.org/10.1016/j.yfpn.2020.01.004
2589-420X/20/

It is now understood that HDP represent independent risk factors for, not simply markers of, future risk for cardiovascular disease [2,5].

Similar to various other factors affecting maternal health, women of color in this country are at an increased risk for developing HDP, as well as several of its major risk factors, such as chronic hypertension and diabetes [3,4,6]. When compared with non-Hispanic white women, non-Hispanic black women are 3.4 times more likely to die as a result of pregnancy-related cardiovascular disease complications [3]. By understanding and intervening in the CHD and CVD cascade, health care providers have the potential to impact longstanding racial disparities in maternal health outcomes in the United States.

Like many other chronic diseases outside pregnancy, the groundwork for most HDP is laid well before signs and symptoms appear: as implantation begins, and before most women are even aware they are pregnant. The stage can be also set by risk factors, which make women physiologically more vulnerable to, and likely to experience, the maladaptations that form the foundation for preeclampsia [2].

By identifying those at increased risk, and mitigating modifiable risk factors before and between pregnancies, there exists the potential to decrease the incidence of HDP, and therefore maternal morbidity and mortality during and beyond pregnancy. By considering pregnancy a "stress test" for life, as well as understanding that preeclampsia is an independent risk factor for cardiovascular disease [2,5], health care providers can better counsel women to undergo targeted screening and help them make decisions and lifestyle modifications that could positively impact their long-term health [3,7].

This article defines HDP, discusses its prevalence, and summarizes the complex cascade, which silently sets the stage for the commonly recognized signs and symptoms of preeclampsia and other HDP. Finally, it addresses implications for primary care providers caring for women before, between, and after their pregnancies.

PREVALENCE OF HYPERTENSION, CARDIOVASCULAR DISEASE, AND HYPERTENSIVE DISORDERS IN PREGNANCY

According to the World Health Organization, CVD is a common affliction for women, with a reported 20% suffering from hypertension and half of all deaths in women attributed to cardiovascular causes [7]. In the United States, it is estimated that coronary artery disease affects 6.1% of women over 20 years of age; a number that increases to more than 20% for women over 75 years [1]. In addition to being responsible for more than 50% of deaths in all women, CVD is the leading cause of mortality in pregnant and postpartum women [1,5]. In non-Hispanic black women in pregnancy, CVD proves to be particularly deadly, with the primary causes of death being attributed to complications related to CVD, preeclampsia, and eclampsia (seizures resulting from preeclampsia). Maternal mortality for non-Hispanic black women is 2 to 3 times that of their white counterparts, even after controls for socioeconomic disparities [6]. Research supports that the increase in maternal deaths due to CVD for all women is from acquired (noncongenital) disease [3].

Chronic hypertension is thought to affect 1% to 2% of all pregnant women, although its incidence is known to be on the increase. Rates of maternal chronic hypertension have increased by 67% in the near decade between 2000 and 2009, with the largest increase, 87%, being among African American women [4]. A discussion of contributing factors, including racism in the health care system and at large, weathering and allostatic load are outside the scope of this article.

Some form of hypertensive disease affects up to 10% of all pregnancies [3]. Estimates of the incidence of preeclampsia vary slightly from source to source, but are thought to range from 2% to 8% [1,2,5] of first pregnancies, with risk in subsequent pregnancies thought to be about 15% [7]. Consistent with rates of other hypertensive disorders, the rate of preeclampsia is also on the increase, with a reported 25% increase in cases of preeclampsia in the United States between 1984 and 2004 [2]. This overall increase in the rate of preeclampsia has been accompanied by an increase in instances of more severe forms of preeclampsia [2].

UNDERSTANDING HYPERTENSIVE DISORDERS IN PREGNANCY

The varied presentation of HDP, including signs and symptoms, severity, timing, and progression, is part of what makes this disease complicated to both diagnose and manage. To combat this difficulty, the American College of Obstetricians and Gynecologists (ACOG) established a task force in 2013, providing clearer definitions to guide both diagnosis and management of HDP. The resultant nomenclature, outlined below, coveys the progressive nature of the disease, which is a shift in understanding for many clinicians [2].

Definitions of hypertensive disorders in pregnancy

Chronic hypertension: raised blood pressure >139/89 predating pregnancy, or before 20 weeks of gestation, or persisting more than 12 weeks postpartum [2]. In patients who have no record of blood pressure before pregnancy, this is at times a retrospective diagnosis. Patients can have preeclampsia superimposed on chronic hypertension. At this time, ACOG has not recommended adoption of American College of Cardiology and the American Heart Association's (AHA) new classification criteria, which would define women with blood pressure 130 to 139/80 to 89 as hypertensive. It may be reasonable to continue any antihypertensive medications for this group of patients and to consider them at increased risk for progressive hypertensive disease, and therefore potential candidates for increased screening during pregnancy [4].

Gestational hypertension: blood pressure greater than 139/89 on 2 separate occasions 4 hours apart after 20 weeks gestation, without signs of preeclampsia or accompanying laboratory abnormalities.

Preeclampsia: blood pressure greater than 139/89 on 2 separate occasions 4 hours apart with other classic signs of preeclampsia: abnormalities in renal function (oliguria, proteinuria, raised blood urea nitrogen and creatinine values), abnormalities in liver function (nausea, vomiting, increased laboratory values), and pulmonary edema.

Preeclampsia can exist either with or without *severe features*. Severe features include: blood pressure greater than 159/109 on 2 separate occasions 4 hours apart, cerebrovascular symptoms (headache, scotomata), pulmonary edema.

Eclampsia: eclamptic seizure resulting from neurologic irritation from preeclampsia.

HELLP: hemolysis, increased liver enzymes, low platelets.

HELLP has traditionally been identified as an end-stage manifestation of pre-eclampsia; however, HELLP can occur without preexisting preeclampsia. Some researchers and clinicians think that a subset of HELLP cases may represent a different pathologic process, which shares many symptomatic features with preeclampsia.

A note on the "20 weeks gestation" threshold: although 20 weeks has been traditionally used as a discerning point for when to consider hypertension chronic versus pregnancy related, there is an acknowledgment that this should not be considered authoritative. Women can present with hypertension that is pregnancy related before 20 weeks, and chronic hypertension can become evident after 20 weeks of gestation, having been masked by normal hemody-namic changes in early pregnancy [4].

Risk factors

Although there are several well-established risk factors for the development of preeclampsia, most preeclampsia occurs in low-risk women in the first preg-nancy [2].

Risk factors include [2]:

- History of preeclampsia
- Age 35 years or older
- African American (moderate risk factor as defined by recommendations for preventative treatment with aspirin, discussed below)
- Chronic hypertension
- Kidney disease
- Obesity, body mass index (BMI) >30
- Lupus and other connective tissue disorders
- Multifetal pregnancy
- Assisted reproductive technology
- Nulliparity
- Diabetes, both gestational and pregestational

Pathophysiology, signs, and symptoms and maternal and fetal consequences of hypertensive disorders of pregnancy

There seem to be several elements at play in the development of preeclampsia. What is not as clear is whether the process is linear, or part of a cyclical phys-iologic process.

Abnormal placentation

In the very early stages of pregnancy, the trophoblast implants in the placental bed and remodels the vasculature to establish a high-flow, low-pressure system that will nurture the fetus for the remainder of the pregnancy. It is known that, in pregnancies affected by preeclampsia, this remodeling of the spiral arteries is impaired. Instead of the formation of a uterine/placental interface that can deliver optimal amounts of oxygenated blood and nutrients to the fetus, the end product is a uterine/placental interface that has restricted flow. This restricted flow happens to varying degrees, explaining why some babies of pre-eclamptic mothers are growth restricted, whereas others are not [2].

The placenta, suffering from ischemia, releases a series of complicated toxins. This release of toxins is the process which gave preeclampsia its former name, toxemia, and is thought to be responsible for causing further down-stream effects (described below).

Imbalance of vasodilating and vasoconstricting agents

Women who have or develop preeclampsia have an enhanced reactivity to angiotensin II, the most potent vasoconstrictor known. The reason for this sensitivity is not well understood. This increased reactivity causes the vessels, including those in the utero-placental bed, to vasoconstrict, leading to the (sometimes intermittent) hallmark hypertension seen in preeclampsia. This vasoconstriction, on the local level, is also thought to cause the headaches and visual changes (blurry vision, scotomata) seen in some women with pre-eclampsia [2].

Release of toxic substance and endothelial damage

Several substances seem to be released by the ischemic placenta as a result of the insult, and these substances exert an effect on the maternal vasculature, leading to endothelial damage (essentially capillary injury and leak). The resultant third spacing is the cause of the edema that is commonly seen with preeclampsia. This "leakiness" can extend to the tubules in the kidneys, resulting in proteinuria. It is also the suspected cause of a less commonly seen symptom of preeclampsia: pulmonary edema or fluid third-spacing into the lungs [2].

Sequelae of preeclampsia

Given this component of the pathophysiology of preeclampsia, it is easy to see why women who have preexisting risk factors for endothelial damage are at increased risk for preeclampsia and for more severe forms of preeclampsia.

By working through the pathophysiology of preeclampsia we have ad-dressed many of the hallmark and diagnostic signs and symptoms: fetal growth restriction (caused by compromised vasculature in the utero-placental bed), hypertension, headache, and visual changes (oversensitivity to angiotensin II leading to vasoconstriction), and edema, proteinuria, and pulmonary edema (capillary leak) [2].

Women with preeclampsia are at risk for several pregnancy-related sequelae, including [3]:

Maternal
- Myocardial infarction [3,4]
- Stroke [3,8]
- Pulmonary edema [2,4]
- Liver dysfunction [2]
- Renal dysfunction [2]
- Disseminated intravascular coagulation [2]
- Eclampsia [2]
- Postpartum hemorrhage [4]

Fetal
- Preterm delivery [2,8]
- Fetal growth restriction [2,8]
- Placental abruption [2,4]
- Intrauterine fetal demise [2,8]

Management of hypertensive disorders in pregnancy

Management of HDP involves a balance of prolonging pregnancy to reduce neonatal health risks associated with prematurity and shortening pregnancy in hopes of minimizing progression of disease and worsening health outcomes for both mother and baby. Management and treatment may include any number of the following [2]:

- Management of blood pressure: balance of maintaining pressure high enough to sustain utero-placental perfusion and low enough to decrease the risk of stroke and other systemic damage. Antihypertensive medications are used to minimize sequelae of preeclampsia and are started if severe range pressures are noted.
- Monitoring for complications when it is in the baby's best interest to remain in utero. This may include increased frequency of maternal visits to monitor for worsening increase in blood pressure or other signs of progression of the disease, or fetal testing.
- Induction of labor: depending on the gestational age, severity of disease, and rate of progression of the symptoms, induction of labor may be undertaken. This is often curative immediately or to within a few days.
- Raising the seizure threshold: induction of labor for women with preeclampsia or gestational hypertension with severe features will likely involve attempts to increase the seizure threshold with administration of intravenous magnesium sulfate.

IMPLICATIONS FOR PRIMARY CARE

Preconception

For women of childbearing age, every primary care encounter is potentially a preconception visit. In addition to addressing medications which may have implications for a pregnancy, it is a time when she may be more motivated to make lifestyle changes that could decrease her risk for HDP and future cardiovascular morbidity. Areas for improvement include those identified by the AHA "Life's Simple 7" campaign [9]:

- Smoking cessation
- Dietary changes
- Increased activity
- Weight loss
- Managing blood pressure
- Controlling cholesterol
- Reducing blood sugar

The American Academy of Family Physicians (AAFP) recommends routine screening for, and implementing lifestyle modifications to mitigate or eliminate, obesity and hypertension during routine primary care encounters [10].

ACOG points to missed opportunities to address cardiovascular risk factors as a contributor to racial health disparities [3]. The preconception period can be a time to optimize identification of risk factors.

Of note, the recommendations for the management of HDP, including timing of delivery, differ depending on the diagnosis of preexisting hypertensive disease. Whether before pregnancy or between pregnancies, it is helpful to obstetric providers when a patient presents with a clear diagnosis regarding preexisting hypertensive disease. Clear communication with women regarding their diagnosis and documentation in the health record allows for more integrated care.

Early pregnancy
Prevention with low-dose aspirin
ACOG and the Society for Maternal-Fetal Medicine (SMFM) support the US Preventative Services Task Force (USPSTF) guidelines for the use of daily low-dose aspirin in high-risk women for prevention of preeclampsia [11]. Aspirin can be used for women with high risk factors (history of preeclampsia, multifetal gestations, renal or autoimmune disease, and chronic hypertension) to reduce the incidence of severe preeclampsia, preterm preeclampsia, and fetal growth restriction [2]. It is also used in women with more than 1 moderate risk factor (first pregnancy, BMI > 30, 35 years or older, family history of preeclampsia, and socioeconomic risk factors, currently poorly defined, and therefore difficult to use as criteria in a meaningful way) for the same reductions [11].

As discussed above, aspirin offers reduction of risk for preeclampsia, intrauterine growth restriction, and need for delivery before 34 and 37 weeks [12]. It may be that one of the main effects is to delay the onset, which in turn mitigates progressive severity of preeclampsia. This initially led to some confusion about whether aspirin use contributes to increased rates of term preeclampsia, as some would-be early presenting cases were converted to late-presenting cases [13].

USPSTF, with the agreement of ACOG and SMFM, recommends daily low-dose aspirin for women with risk factors for preeclampsia starting before 16 weeks of gestation, ideally at 12 weeks, and continuing through delivery [11].

Postpartum

The postpartum time, typically defined as the 6 weeks after delivery, is one of increased risk for morbidity and mortality related to cardiovascular disease [3], and it is important to be aware that this risk extends beyond what is typically seen as the postpartum period. Most morbidity and mortality related to cardiovascular disease in postpartum women occurs more than 42 days after delivery [3]. This is a time when women are more likely to present to primary care and nonobstetric emergency settings because they consider the pregnancy and its related risk to be in the past. A simple question included in the medical history about having given birth within the previous year can elicit information about this time of increased risk.

It is essential that postpartum patients be aware of the signs and symptoms of preeclampsia after delivery. Among women who present in the postpartum period with eclampsia or stroke, many have had symptoms for at least hours and sometimes days before presentation [2].

In the postpartum setting, any increase in blood pressure should be immediately evaluated for HDP. Any chest pain or other potential cardiac symptoms, including shortness of breath, vomiting, reflux, or diaphoresis, should be triaged as if they could have a cardiac cause [3].

Some sources suggest that better identification of cardiac sources of abnormal symptoms in pregnancy and postpartum could lead to a 25% reduction in maternal death [3].

Primary care clinicians should also be aware of commonly prescribed medications that can impact blood pressure issues postpartum. A prime example is nonsteroidal anti-inflammatory drugs (NSAIDs), which are commonly used in the postpartum period for pain control. NSAIDs decrease prostaglandins, leading to sodium retention and inhibition of vasodilatation, which can cause an increase in blood pressure. This being said, it is important that opioids not be considered a simple default option for pain management [4].

Breastfeeding should be recommended and supported, given the cardiometabolic benefits to mothers, in addition to benefits for baby [3]. Breastfeeding has been found to decrease future risk of type 2 diabetes, obesity, and hypertension [14].

Beyond postpartum

It has been established that women with preeclampsia are at increased risk for HDP in future pregnancies, and even more so if they experienced severe or early-onset disease.

Outside of pregnancy, women with preeclampsia have an almost doubled risk for cardiovascular diseases, including hypertension, myocardial infarction and congestive heart failure, stroke, and cardiovascular mortality, later in life [1,2,8,12]. It seems that preeclampsia is an independent risk factor, not simply a marker, for CVD [5]. Only approximately half of future risk seems to be related to risk factors that existed before pregnancy [2,8]. Likely because of the resultant endothelial damage, preeclampsia in and of itself affects long-term cardiovascular health [2,5]. In addition, women with recurrent preeclampsia, especially early onset or severe preeclampsia, are at an even higher lifetime risk [1–3,7,8,12].

In terms of other disease processes, women with a history of preeclampsia have an almost 2-fold increased risk of developing diabetes outside of pregnancy [1] and a relative risk of at least 4.7 times of developing end-stage renal disease [3,8,12]. History of HDP should be noted in the patient's medical record, and plans made for continued testing and monitoring (see later discussion).

Pharmacologic management
After birth, women with prepregnancy chronic hypertension should continue their antihypertensive medication, but will need adjustment in dosage to adjust for the decrease in blood volume and glomerular filtration rate that take place after delivery. This can be done by or in consultation with the patient's obstetric provider [8].

After birth, women with gestational hypertension or preeclampsia with severe features may remain on antihypertensives for some time if needed to control blood pressures. Little guidance exists on when and how to discontinue medications, although it is clear that it should be done under the guidance of a health care provider. Because many women stop seeing their obstetric providers within 6 to 8 weeks after completion of pregnancy, decision-making on when to stop antihypertensive medications may fall to the primary care clinician.

All women with chronic hypertension or any HDP must be monitored for the development of postpartum preeclampsia [8].

Interventions
Several sources recommend routine screening for, and intervention around, cardiovascular health in the time after a pregnancy [1,3,8].

ACOG recommends a "3 month comprehensive cardiovascular postpartum visit," which would include an individualized plan and could happen in the obstetric or primary care setting. Such a visit would include a history of pertinent symptoms, physical examination, assessment of BMI and waist circumference, and measurement of vital signs (including blood pressure, heart rate, respiratory rate, and oxygen saturation). Fasting blood glucose or hemoglobin A1C and a complete lipid panel should also be considered [3]. Although this visit may be done by the obstetric care team, this standard is far from routine and primary care providers may be charged with taking the lead on this follow-up.

AHA argues "it is reasonable to (1) consider evaluating all women starting 6 months to 1 year postpartum, as well as those who are past childbearing age, for a history of preeclampsia/eclampsia and document their history of preeclampsia/eclampsia as a risk factor and (2) evaluate and treat for cardiovascular risk factors including hypertension, obesity, smoking, and dyslipidemia" [8].

Primary care clinicians should use cardiovascular risk assessment tools to guide counseling and management of patients, keeping in mind that not all tools will consider HDP a risk factor, despite supporting evidence. In their 2013 Guideline for the Prevention of Stroke in Women, AHA lists preeclampsia as a risk factor for stroke [8].

According to estimates in 1 study, lifestyle interventions for women with a history of preeclampsia could lead to a decrease in CVD of 4% to 13% [5].

ACOG further argues that women with borderline blood pressure or lipid screening should have testing repeated after 6 to 12 months of lifestyle modifications [3].

SUMMARY

The impact of CVD on women's health worldwide is significant and increasing. HDP is a risk factor for, and contributor to, lifelong CVD risk. Alongside rates of CVD, HDP are on the increase. By understanding risk factors, identifying women at risk, and counseling around screening and lifestyle modifications to decrease risk, health care providers can potentially decrease the incidence and impact of CVD. Given the stark reality of racial disparities in maternal morbidity and mortality in one of the most advanced health care systems in the world, providers are also poised to close the persistent and shameful gap that exists between outcomes for women and babies of color and their white counterparts.

References

[1] Ahmed R, Dunford J, Mehran R, et al. Pre-eclampsia and future cardiovascular risk among women: a review. J Am Coll Cardiol 2014;63:1815–22.

[2] ACOG. Practice bulletin number 202: gestational hypertension and preeclampsia. Obstet Gynecol 2019;133(1):e1–25.

[3] ACOG. Practice bulletin number 212: pregnancy and heart disease. Obstet Gynecol 2019;133(5):e320–56.

[4] ACOG. Practice bulletin number 203: chronic hypertension in pregnancy. Obstet Gynecol 2019;133(1):e26–50.

[5] Berks D, Hoedjes M, Raat H, et al. Risk of cardiovascular disease after pre-eclampsia and the effect of lifestyle interventions : a literature-based study. BJOG 2013;120(8):924–31.

[6] US Department of Health and Human Services/Centers for Disease Control and Prevention, Petersen EE, Davis NL, Goodman D, et al. Racial/ethnic disparities in pregnancy-related deaths—United States, 2007–2016. MMWR Morb Mortal Wkly Rep 2019;68(35): 762–5.

[7] Brouwers L, van derMeiden-van Roest AJ, Savelkoul C, et al. Recurrence of pre-eclampsia and the risk of future hypertension and cardiovascular disease: a systemic review and meta-analysis. BJOG 2018;125(13):1642–54.

[8] Bushnell C, McCullough LD. AHA/ASA guideline: guidelines for the prevention of stroke in women: a statement for healthcare professionals from the American Heart Association/ American Stroke Association. Stroke 2014;45:1545–88.

[9] American Heart Association. Available at: https://www.heart.org/en/professional/workplace-health/lifes-simple-7. Accessed October 12, 2019.

[10] AAFP. Preconception care (position paper). Available at: https://www.aafp.org/about/policies/all/preconception-care.html#References. Accessed November 9, 2019.

[11] ACOG and SMFM. ACOG committee opinion no. 743: low-dose aspirin use during pregnancy. Obstet Gynecol 2018;132(1):e44–52.

[12] Resnik R, Lockwood CJ, Moore T, et al, editors. Creasy and Resnik's maternal-fetal medicine: principles and practice. Philadephia: Elsevier; 2019.

[13] Wright D, Nicolaides KH. Aspirin delays development of preeclampsia. Am J Obstet Gynecol 2019;220:580.e1-6.
[14] Perrine C, Nelson J, Corbelli J, et al. Lactation and maternal cardio-metabolic health. Annu Rev Nutr 2016;36:627–45.

Advances in Family Practice Nursing 2 (2020) 115–124

ADVANCES IN FAMILY PRACTICE NURSING

ELSEVIER
MOSBY

Caring for Women with Circumcision

A Primary Care Perspective

Carol Cathleen Ziegler, MSN, DNP, APRN, NP-C*,
Geri C. Reeves, MSN, PhD, APRN, FNP-BC

Vanderbilt University School of Nursing, 461 21st Avenue South, Nashville, TN 37240, USA

Keywords
- Female genital mutilation • Female circumcision • Female genital cutting
- Infibulation • Deinfibulation

Key points
- Primary care providers should be prepared to provide patient-centered, culturally sensitive care for women with female genital mutilation (FGM) and ensure that a qualified medical interpreter is present if necessary, preferably female.
- Primary care providers should be able to identify patients at risk for FGM, identify FGM by type, and clearly document presence of FGM and any related complications in the medical record.
- Long-term complications related to FGM presenting in primary care include chronic pain, scarring, sexual dysfunction, vaginal and urinary tract infections, urinary retention, menstrual complications, and psychological symptoms.
- All women with FGM should be offered counseling for possible mental health consequences related to trauma, and women with FGM type 3 (infibulation) should be offered referral for deinfibulation.
- Women with FGM should be offered mental health services, screenings for sexually transmitted infections, cervical cancer, human immunodeficiency virus, hepatitis, as well as the human papilloma virus vaccine according to the most up-to-date guidelines.

INTRODUCTION

According to the World Health Organization (WHO), more than 200 million girls and women alive now have been subjected to female genital mutilation

*Corresponding author. E-mail address: Carol.c.ziegler@vanderbilt.edu

https://doi.org/10.1016/j.yfpn.2020.01.005

(FGM) [1]. The procedure is mostly performed on young girls between infancy and 15 years of age [1]. Three million girls continue to be at risk for FGM annually [2]. FGM is prevalent in 30 countries in Africa and in parts of Asia and the Middle East [1]. Although FGM is most prevalent in sub-Saharan Africa, global migration patterns have increased the risk of FGM among women and girls living in high-income countries, including the United States. In 2013, there were up to 507,000 US women and girls who had undergone FGM in their home countries or in communities in the United States or were at risk of being subjected to the procedure in the United States [2]. In the year 2000, the same estimate was 228,000 [3]. The rapid increase in women and girls at risk reflects an increase in immigration to the United States. The number of women and girls at risk for FGM varies across states [2]. According to the Population Reference Bureau, in 2013, approximately three-fifths of all women and girls at risk of FGM/female genital cutting (FGC) lived in 8 states: California, Maryland, Minnesota, New Jersey, New York, Texas, Virginia, and Washington. California had the largest at-risk population (57,000), followed by New York (48,000) and Minnesota (44,000) [3]. Although the population at risk is still highly concentrated in large entryway states, many immigrant families have fanned out from traditional immigrant entry states to new destinations around the country [2]. However, clinicians should not assume that a woman from a country practicing FGM has undergone the procedure or that all women who have undergone FGM have complications. Clinicians should keep in mind that, until the feminist movement, FGM types 1and 2 were performed in the United States by medical doctors for such prefeminist diagnoses as frigidity, hysteria, melancholia, and nymphomania, and were even covered by insurance until 1977 [4]. Many Western women now undergo body "enhancement" through female genital cosmetic surgery, which is marketed as a way to enhance women's appearance or sexual function and is not medically indicated, and also not well researched regarding safety and long-term complications [5].

DEFINITIONS AND A BRIEF BACKGROUND

FGM/FGC is defined by the WHO as any procedure involving partial or total removal of the external female genitalia or other injury to the female genital organs for nonmedical reasons [6]. Many terms have been used to describe the practice. The WHO uses the term FGM, and other organizations use the more neutral term female genital cutting or female genital alteration [6]. This article uses the term FGM. The WHO classifies the procedure into 4 major types. See Table 1 for a description of procedures.

ACCESS TO CARE: PROVIDER COMMUNICATION

Aside from the domestic medical screening evaluation required of immigrants and refugees at the time of immigration or resettlement, the episodic encounter at a family practice clinic may be a woman's first interaction with her new health care environment. It is well established in the literature that there are

Table 1
Descriptions of procedures for female genital mutilation

Type 1	Often referred to as clitoridectomy, this is the partial or total removal of the clitoris (a small, sensitive, and erectile part of the female genitals), and, in very rare cases, only the prepuce (the fold of skin surrounding the clitoris)
Type 2	Often referred to as excision, this is the partial or total removal of the clitoris and the labia minora (the inner folds of the vulva), with or without excision of the labia majora (the outer folds of skin of the vulva)
Type 3	Often referred to as infibulation, this is the narrowing of the vaginal opening through the creation of a covering seal. The seal is formed by cutting and repositioning the labia minora, or labia majora, sometimes through stitching, with or without removal of the clitoris (clitoridectomy)
Type 4	All other harmful procedures to the female genitalia for nonmedical purposes; eg, pricking, piercing, incising, scraping, and cauterizing the genital area

Data from World Health Organization. Female Genital Mutilation. 31 Janaury 2018. Available at: https://www.who.int/news-room/fact-sheets/detail/female-genital-mutilation.

significant knowledge gaps among clinicians when it comes to caring for women with FGM [7], and provider discomfort discussing FGM negatively affects the health care experiences of women, increasing feelings of helplessness, vulnerability, anxiety, and uncertainty [7]. Provider discomfort and reluctance to discuss FGM, and the cultural taboo women may feel in speaking about the practice, create a double silence [8]. Open communication may be further impeded by language barriers and cultural insensitivity of the provider, exacerbating reluctance to seek health care and further diminishing health care access for this population [8].

Providers must work closely with patients and communities to build trust and ensure that patients enjoy a welcoming clinical environment. Ensure access to a certified medical interpreter, preferably female, if language barriers are present, because research indicates that because this is a culturally sensitive and gender-specific issue, many women with FGM prefer female interpreters [9]. It is recommended to use medically certified interpreters, not family members, and to ensure that the woman is comfortable with the interpreter and that the interpreter does not support the practice of FGM [9]. Document the presence of the medical interpreter in the medical record. Although the WHO does recommend using the term FGM in clinical settings among professionals, many patients understandably find the term offensive, so in the patient encounter it is preferred to use female circumcision, but, ideally, use the term the patient prefers [10]. A list of traditional terms by country for FGM was created by the FGM Center and may be accessed at https://www.28toomany.org/static/media/uploads/Country%20Images/PDF/fgm-terminology_nat_fgm_centre.pdf. This list may be shared with patients at the time of the visit, facilitating discussion of FGM and allowing patients the opportunity to inform their providers of

their preferences. A world map may be displayed in the office and allows her to indicate to you where she is from and facilitate the discussion around FGM. In addition, providers may use an image of the different types of FGM so that a woman can inform the provider regarding the type of FGM she experienced before the examination. Hearst and Molnar [10] include in their article an image, which may be accessed online at https://www.mayoclinicproceedings.org/article/S0025-6196(13)00264-4/fulltext#appsec1. Another excellent resource for providers with visual references for FGM types was developed by Abdulcadir and colleagues [11] and may be accessed at https://journals.lww.com/greenjournal/Fulltext/2016/11000/
Female_Genital_Mutilation__A_Visual_Reference_and.4.aspx.

Ultimately, provider comfort with discussing FGM improves the patient experience and creates the foundation for a trusting relationship, decreasing significant barriers to care for this at-risk population. Box 1 summarizes key points for communication.

TAKING THE HISTORY

The most common conditions encountered in the family practice clinic attributable to long-term complications from FGM may be grouped into disorders related to chronic vulvar or pelvic pain, cysts and keloids related to tissue scarring, sexual dysfunction, vaginal and urinary tract infections (UTIs), urinary retention, menstrual complications, and psychological symptoms related to the trauma of FGM [10,12–14]. Evaluation and management of these conditions are discussed later, with up-to-date clinical recommendations where appropriate. Women seeking primary care for episodic complaints or preventive visits are likely to be presenting with long-term complications caused by FGM types 1, 2, and 3, because short-term complications would have occurred at the time the cutting took place and are often severe, including bleeding, infection, and death [13–15]. Women who have experienced FGM type 3 are at greatest risk for more severe long-term complications [12–14]. Also, some women who have experienced FGM do not experience complications and

---

Box 1: Key points for communication with patients with female genital mutilation

1. Ensure the office environment is welcoming
2. Ensure a female medical interpreter is present and that the patient feels comfortable with the interpreter if language barriers exist
3. Ensure that the interpreter does not support FGM
4. When referring to FGM, use terminology that the patient prefers
5. Use a trauma-informed care approach at all times
6. Conduct the history and education with patient sitting upright and clothed
7. Always respect patient privacy, confidentiality, and autonomy

therefore it is critical that providers pay close attention to the patient's concerns and feelings about her FGM status.

If FGM status is unknown at the time of the visit, the provider should consider risk factors for FGM in adult women, which include immigrant or refugee status from a country or community known to practice FGM, or the presence of a first-degree or second-degree female relative with presence of FGM. Of note, if a provider is seeing a minor who has not experienced FGM and risk factors for FGM are present, or if the provider is seeing a minor with FGM and the timeline indicates that the FGM occurred after the minor's arrival in the United States, the provider should be alerted to risk for FGM to be performed on the child or the potential risk for vacation cutting, respectively. Vacation cutting occurs when families travel to their home countries for the purpose of having their daughters undergo FGM. In this case, child protective services should be notified and the family should be informed that FGM on minors, including vacation cutting, is illegal in the United States.

When taking the history, be sure to assess obstetric and menstrual history. The presence of FGM is assessed during the surgical or obstetric history or just before performing a pelvic examination. Providers should use inclusive, nonjudgmental language, such as, "Some women from your community have experienced genital cutting or circumcision. Have you experienced this?" Hearst and Molnar [10] include a table with guidelines for discussing FGM with patients. If the woman affirms the presence of genital cutting, she can be shown a list of terms and also a picture so she can inform you of the term she prefers and the type and degree of her status.

When the condition is identified, the provider should document the type of FGM present (see Table 1). During this evaluation, it is crucial that women are informed that the practice is illegal in the United States and given resources and referral for psychological counseling if desired. As mentioned previously, if patients have female children, inform them that FGM is illegal in the United States and that vacation cutting requires mandatory reporting. Be aware that refugees from conflict zones may also have experienced sexual trauma and rape, so inquire about any history of trauma or violence, sexual abuse, or rape. Clinicians should consistently use a trauma-informed care approach on all patients with a history of FGM [16]. Conduct the patient history and patient education with the patient sitting upright and fully clothed and be sure to carefully explain all components of examination and obtain verbal consent. Complete a review of systems and history of present illness if the patient is presenting with a chief complaint. Many women with FGM are unaware of the link between the practice and health complications, so inquire about the most common symptoms related to long-term complications of FGM, including pelvic/abdominal pain, pain with sexual activity, genital scarring, difficulty with menstruation or urination, painful menstruation or urination, and any vaginal lesions, discharge, or odor that she is concerned about or concern for sexually transmitted infections. Assess for symptoms of anxiety, depression, somatization, and posttraumatic stress. Assess her sexual satisfaction level and her

personal safety, because some women with FGM experience lower sexual pleasure because of pain and also may be at risk for intimate partner violence
[13,14,17].

DIAGNOSIS AND MANAGEMENT OF LONG-TERM COMPLICATIONS RELATED TO FEMALE GENITAL MUTILATION

Based on the patient's presenting complaint, a pelvic examination or visual inspection may be indicated. Explain that you will conduct a genital examination
and tell her what you are going to do before you begin [18]. Ask the patient
which position she is most comfortable in and ensure that she is covered
and draped appropriately [18]. If a pelvic examination is indicated, use the
smallest speculum possible and ensure that the last three-quarters of the speculum blade is well lubricated. Inform the patient that if at any time she experiences pain, or wants to stop the examination, her wish will be honored.
Patients with presenting gynecologic complaints that cannot tolerate an examination because of discomfort, likely with FGM type 3, should be referred to a
specialist for evaluation.

Pain

Women who have experienced FGM may present with chronic or acute vulvar
or pelvic pain, which may range from mild to severe and may interfere with
their sexual pleasure and quality of life [13,19]. Although FGM type 3 often results in the most severe complications, women with FGM types 1 and 2 may
also present with issues related to pain. Chronic pelvic pain is defined as
pain in the abdomen, pelvis, or low back lasting more than 6 months and often
most noted during sexual activity. On visual inspection, note the type and degree of FGM, presence of any visible scarring, keloids, or epidermal inclusion
cysts. If painless cysts, scarring, or keloids are present and abscess is ruled out,
reassure the patient that treatment is not needed but that she may be referred
for surgery if the lesion is emotionally or psychologically upsetting for her
[10,19]. Assess for tenderness to palpation of the vulva and vaginal opening.
Perform urinalysis to eliminate urinary UTI as a possible cause and complete
a pelvic examination and sexually transmitted infection screen to rule out pelvic inflammatory disease and uterine fibroids. Ultrasonography assists in ruling
out uterine issues such as fibroids as a cause and provides an indication for
referral if ovarian cysts, endometriosis, or endometrial thickening are present.
Patients with chronic pelvic pain not caused by infection should be referred to
women's health or gynecology. If underlying causes are ruled out, the patient
may be treated with nonsteroidal antiinflammatory drugs (NSAIDs) and also
advised to take measures to make sexual activity more comfortable, such as
use of water-based lubricants, and positioning. Patients with vulvodynia, irritation, and pain of the vulva with intercourse may be advised to use water-based
lubricants during intercourse, wear all-cotton underwear, and avoid using any
scented or nonhypoallergenic products on the area. Vulvar vestibulitis is suspected if the pain is reproduced with contact with a moist cotton swab along

a narrow band of tissue just outside the vaginal opening [13]. Clitoral neuroma is suspected if the patient reports exquisite pain with light touch with a cotton swab around the clitoral area on examination [20,21]. Although there is no direct consensus evidence available on management strategies for vulvodynia, vulvar vestibulitis, and clitoral pain in these women, use of a water-soluble lubricant with sexual intercourse, avoiding activities that exacerbate pain, wearing loose-fitting cotton underwear to avoid friction, and use of local topical anesthetics such as lidocaine cream may help decrease pain [21]. Surgical correction may be indicated in women with clitoral neuroma, but evidence is unclear as to long-term success [10]. If, on visual inspection and examination, no apparent cause of pain is identified, and supportive care does not relieve the pain, refer to women's health or gynecology.

Sexual concerns
Women with FGM may experience dyspareunia, anorgasmia, and decreased enjoyment of sexual activity. Causes may be physical, related to scarring, vaginal dryness caused by excision of glands from FGM, or removal of the clitoris and pain caused by infibulation. Psychological trauma from FGM also affects sexual health [13–15,19]. If use of water-based lubricants to combat vaginal dryness or positional changes does not relieve pain with sex, refer her to gynecology. If she has FGM type 3, discuss deinfibulation with her and refer her to gynecology. All women with sexual symptoms related to FGM that are not alleviated with the interventions mentioned should be referred to gynecology or women's health and also offered sexual or psychological counseling [19].

Vaginal infections
Although it does not seem that FGM increases a woman's risk for gonorrhea, chlamydia, trichomoniasis, or pelvic inflammatory disease, FGM does seem to increase the risk for bacterial vaginosis, vaginal candidiasis, and herpes simplex virus [10] and it is thought that scarring, especially with infibulation, is a possible cause [10]. If left untreated, vaginal infections may progress to pelvic inflammatory disease. Women with FGM presenting with complaints raising suspicion for vaginal infections should be tested and managed according to guidelines for the relevant infection. If infections are recurrent and obstructive scarring is present, offer the patient referral for surgical management and provide patient education on symptomatic management and hygiene practices in addition to evidence-based pharmacologic therapy. Because of potential barriers to receiving up-to-date cervical cancer screenings, providers should offer the human papilloma virus vaccine.

Urinary complications (infections and anatomic complications)
FGM type 3 increases risk for UTIs when urinary flow is obstructed because of infibulation or scarring [10,13,19]. Women presenting with urinary complaints should receive urinalysis to rule out UTI and clinicians should assess for pyelonephritis. Urine culture and sensitivity should be obtained if frequency of UTIs indicates a complicated UTI or recurrent UTI or if the patient was recently

treated with antibiotics. Supportive care and evidence-based pharmacologic therapy should be initiated with positive urinalysis. Patients should be offered referral for deinfibulation if they are experiencing recurrent UTIs and have a history of FGM type 3 [10,13,19]. In the absence of a positive urinalysis, painful or difficult urination raises suspicion for urinary retention or obstruction in this population. Assess the patient for incomplete emptying of the bladder and also for incontinence. If obstruction or retention is suspected, refer the patient to gynecology [10,13,19].

Menstrual complications

Women with FGM type 3 may experience secondary dysmenorrhea from scarring or infibulation that impedes the passing of menstrual blood, resulting in accumulation of blood within the uterus and/or vagina [13]. It may be difficult to conduct a pelvic examination on a woman experiencing this degree of complication from scarring or infibulation, so referral to gynecology for deinfibulation is indicated [10,13,19]. For menstrual pain not related to infibulation, patients may be managed with NSAIDs or oral contraceptives.

MENTAL HEALTH

Patients that have experienced FGM are often either immigrants who have chosen to resettle in a new environment or refugees who may have experienced severe civil conflict. Although both groups may have history of trauma and psychological consequences related to the practice and experience of FGM, refugee patients may have higher incidence of posttraumatic stress disorder and psychological consequences caused by the conditions surrounding their displacement and the stress of the new environment [12,13,16]. Management of the psychological sequelae of FGM should include assessments for depression, anxiety, and posttraumatic stress disorder, and all patients should be offered psychological counseling and treatment of any underlying mental health conditions [12,19]. It is important to remember that, in the context of these complex factors, many women have psychological trauma and mental health concerns unrelated to FGM. Access to appropriate mental health services is a challenge in many communities and linguistic barriers that necessitate using interpreters in psychotherapy does dramatically alter the dyadic therapeutic relationship [22]. In addition, many women who have undergone FGM have had positive experiences and feelings related to the practice and may not have any trauma or psychological sequela from the experience. Providers should assess how the woman feels about her own body and experiences and proceed based on her desires and specific needs.

SUMMARY AND IMPLICATIONS FOR PRACTICE

In 2016, the WHO released guidelines for the care of women with FGM [19]. The summary may be accessed at https://www.who.int/reproductivehealth/topics/fgm/management-health-complications-fgm/en/

The following is a bulleted summary of the guidelines that relate to the primary care topics discussed in this article:

- Offer information, education, and communication to all women with FGM.
- Offer deinfibulation to all women with FGM type 3.
- All women who have experienced FGM and experience psychological symptoms should be offered cognitive behavior therapy and psychological counseling services.
- Women should be offered screening for sexually transmitted infections, human immunodeficiency virus, and hepatitis B and C.
- Women experiencing sexual dysfunction should be offered sexual counseling and treatment/referral for any underlying issues.
- Women experiencing urologic complications, recurrent UTIs, or urinary retention should be offered surgical correction/deinfibulation.

Primary care providers are on the frontlines of communities and are key advocates for at-risk populations. Because of linguistic, logistical, cultural, and sociologic barriers, many women with FGM experience isolation, vulnerability, and diminished access to health care, and are at increased risk for poor health outcomes and decreased quality of life. Many have experienced extreme trauma and are unsure how to navigate the US health care system, and they may lack the financial and social resources to do so successfully. Primary care clinicians are well positioned to provide education on general health as well as health implications of FGM, and build relationships and trust over time, improving access to care for this at-risk population.

Disclosure

The authors have nothing to disclose.

References

[1] World Health Organization. Female genital mutilation. 2018. Available at: https://www.who.int. Accessed August 26, 2019.

[2] Mather M, Feldman-Jacobs C. Women and girls at risk of female genital mutilation/cutting in the US. 2016. Available at: https://www.prb.org/us-fgmc/#. Accessed August 26, 2019.

[3] Brigham and Women's Hospital. Female genital cutting research. Available at: https://www.brighamandwomens.org/Departments_and_Services/obgyn/services/africanwomenscenter/research.aspx. Accessed September 3, 2019.

[4] Webber S, Schonfeld T. Cutting history, cutting culture: female circumcision in the United States. Am J Bioeth 2003;3(2):65-6.

[5] Cain J, Iglesia C, Dickens B, et al. Body enhancement through female genital cosmetic surgery creates ethical and rights dilemmas. Int J Gynaecol Obstet 2013;122:169-72.

[6] Puppo V. Female genital mutilation and cutting: an anatomical review and alternative rites. Clin Anat 2017;30:81-8.

[7] Smith H, Stein K. Health information interventions for female genital mutilation. Int J Gynaecol Obstet 2017;136(Suppl 1):79-82.

[8] Evans C, Tweheyo R, McGarry J, et al. Seeking culturally safe care: a qualitative systematic review of the healthcare experiences of women and girls who have undergone female genital mutilation/cutting. BMJ Open 2019;9:e027452.

[9] Jordal M, Wahlberg A. Challenges in providing quality care for women with female genital cutting in sweden – a literature review. Sex Reprod Healthc 2018;17:91-6.

[10] Hearst A, Molnar A. Female genital cutting: an evidence-based approach to clinical management for the primary care physician. Mayo Clin Proc 2013;88(6):618–29.

[11] Abdulcadir J, Catania L, Hindin M, et al. Female genital mutilation: a visual reference and learning tool for health care professionals. Obstet Gynecol 2016;128(5):958–63.

[12] von Rege I, Campion D. Female genital mutilation: implications for clinical practice. Br J Nurs 2017;26(18):s22–7.

[13] Toubia N. Caring for women with circumcision: a technical manual for health care providers. New York: Research, Action, and Information Network for Bodily Integrity of Women (RAINBO); 1999.

[14] Toubia N. Female circumcision as a public health issue. N Engl J Med 1994;331:712–6.

[15] WHO. Health risks of female genital mutilation. Available at: https://www.who.int/reproductivehealth/topics/fgm/health_consequences_fgm/en/. Accessed August 30, 2019.

[16] Lever H, Ottenheimer D, Teysir J, et al. Depression, anxiety, post-traumatic stress disorder and a history of pervasive gender-based violence among women asylum seekers who have undergone female genital mutilation/cutting: a retrospective case review. J Immigr Minor Health 2019;21(3):483–9.

[17] Salihu H, August E, Salemi J, et al. The association between female genital mutilation and intimate partner violence. BJOG 2012;119(13):1597–605.

[18] Bates C, Carroll N, Potter J. The challenging pelvic exam. J Gen Intern Med 2011;26(6): 651–7.

[19] World Health Organization. WHO guidelines on the management of health complications from female genital mutilation. Geneva (Switzerland): WHO; 2016. Available at: http://www.who.int/reproductivehealth/topics/fgm/management-health-complications-fgm/en/.

[20] Rouzi A. Epidermal clitoral inclusion cysts: not a rare complication of female genital mutilation. Hum Reprod 2010;25(7):1672–4.

[21] Zoorob D, Kristinsdottir K, Klein T, et al. Case report: symptomatic clitoral neuroma within an epidermal inclusion cyst at the site of prior female genital cutting. Case Rep Obstet Gynecol 2019;2019:5347873.

[22] Miller K, Martell Z, Pazdirek L. The role of interpreters in psychotherapy with refugees: an exploratory study. Am J Orthopsychiatry 2005;75(1):27–39.

Advances in Family Practice Nursing 2 (2020) 125–143

ADVANCES IN FAMILY PRACTICE NURSING

Insomnia Treatment in the Primary Care Setting

Jennifer G. Hensley, EdD, CNM, WHNP-BC, LCCE[a],*,
Janet R. Beardsley, DNP, CNM, ANP-C[b,c,1]

[a]Baylor University, Louise Herrington School of Nursing, 333 North Washington Avenue, Dallas, TX 75246, USA; [b]Winthrop Family Medicine, 16 Commerce Plaza, Suite 3A, Winthrop, ME 04364, USA; [c]MaineGeneral Health, Augusta, ME, USA

Keywords
- Insomnia • Healthy sleep • Daytime impairment • Cognitive behavioral therapy
- Sleep restriction • Sleep diary • Sleep hygiene

Key points
- Initial evaluation and treatment of acute and chronic insomnia can be handled by clinicians in the primary care setting.
- Lack of sleep associated with insomnia symptoms can lead to daytime impairments.
- Cognitive behavioral therapy and sleep restriction therapy are the proven effective treatments for insomnia.
- Treatment goals include improvement in the quality of sleep and lessening of daytime impairments.
- Insomnia can be exacerbated by, or exacerbate, medical and psychiatric comorbidities.

INTRODUCTION

Insomnia is one of the most common sleep complaints in the adult population [1,2]. Primary care clinicians often lack the time and resources to address insomnia, thereby providing basic education about sleep hygiene and suggestions for over-the-counter sleep aids, or ordering a hypnotic. Sleep hygiene alone, with or without a medication or supplement, may not help the patient as there is more than one type of insomnia, and insomnia is often

---

[1]Present address: 43 York Road. Minot. ME 04258.

*Corresponding author. E-mail address: jennifer_hensley@baylor.edu

https://doi.org/10.1016/j.yfpn.2020.01.012
2589-420X/20/

multifactorial. This article is written to help primary care clinicians evaluate insomnia complaints, recommend first-line treatment, and identify when to refer to a sleep medicine specialist.

The prevalence of insomnia is difficult to determine, as varying definitions have been used in population-based study designs. Attempts to approximate the prevalence in developed countries estimate chronic insomnia in the adult population at 10% [3], increasing to 50% when acute insomnia is included [4]. Patients who have medical and/or psychiatric comorbidities increase the prevalence of insomnia to 50% to 75% [5].

Sleep loss related to insomnia causes not only sleepiness, but personal distress, irritability, discord in relationships, daytime impairment, lost hours and days at work, and worsening medical conditions [1]. In 2006, the Institute of Medicine (now the National Academy of Medicine) recommended better public awareness of inadequate sleep, its consequences, as well as increased clinician skill related to diagnosis and treatment of sleep disorders [6].

WHY SLEEP?

Although the actual role of sleep is incompletely understood, it is necessary for memory consolidation, restoration and rejuvenation of physiologic processes that lead to physical health and optimal immune function, as well as good mental health and clear cognition [7]. The recommendation for adults to achieve adequate sleep is at least 7 hours per night on a routine basis [8]. Sleeping longer than 9 hours per night seems to have no benefit for most individuals [8,9]. In fact, a slightly higher risk of overall mortality exists for adults who sleep less than 7 hours or more than 9 hours per night (relative risk [RR] = 1.0; 95% CI, 1.06–1.15 and RR = 1.23; 95% CI, 1.17–1.30, respectively) [10]. Actual time asleep should match the timing of a patient's circadian rhythm and propensity for sleep. The "average" patient will require between 7 and 8 hours of sleep per night between 10 PM and 6 AM, but circadian rhythm differences exist. Not every patient is average when it comes to sleeping, and the clinician must query as to preferences and needs. The "owl" prefers to fall asleep and rise later (eg, 1 AM to 9 AM), whereas the "lark" prefers earlier sleep and rise times (eg, 8 PM to 4 AM). In addition, there are individuals who require longer and shorter sleep periods than 7 to 8 hours per night. There are those who require 9 to 10 hours (long sleepers) and those who require 6 hours of sleep or less (short sleepers) per night [11]. The best way to ascertain individual preferences and needs is to ask, *"When you are on vacation, what are your preferred bedtimes and hours of sleep?"* Fig. 1 represents life demands that impact individual sleep need differences.

Healthy sleep does not have an absolute definition as it is largely subjective. When a patient presents complaining of fatigue or sleepiness during the day, assessing their sleep should be a first step. To ask a patient about their subjective experience of sleep in a minute, the acronym "SATED" is a useful tool [12]. Negative responses are an opportunity to ask the patient more targeted

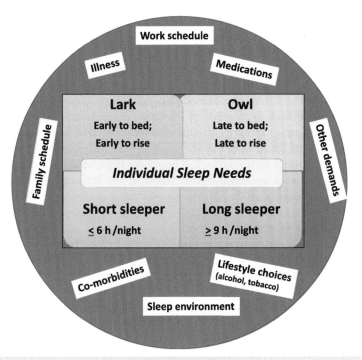

Fig. 1. Individual sleep needs.

questions about sleep that could be related to a sleep disorder. Work and life schedules factor into what the patient experiences as insomnia. If a patient does not (or cannot) set aside 7 to 8 hours per night for sleep, then the problem is not insomnia, it is a problem with scheduling. In this case, cognitive behavioral therapy and hypnotics will not be helpful. Addressing sleep satisfaction in primary care is important for both short-term and long-term physical and emotional health (Table 1).

Table 1	
SATED	
S – Are you SATISFIED with your sleep?	Subjective sense of well-being
A – Are you ALERT during the waking hours?	No falling asleep at work or while driving; no need for napping during the day
T – Is the TIMING of your sleep appropriate?	Going to bed when tired, getting out of bed in the morning without difficulty
E – Is your sleep EFFICIENT?	Staying asleep 85% of the time in bed
D – Is the DURATION for sleep adequate?	Do you have 7–8 h to devote to uninterrupted sleep?

Data from Buysse DJ. Sleep health: can we define it? Does it matter? Sleep 2014;37(1):9-17 [12].

DEFINITION OF INSOMNIA

In the 2014 International Classification of Sleep Disorders 3rd Edition, insomnia is defined as a "…1. persistent difficulty with sleep initiation, duration, consolidation, or quality, 2. that occurs despite adequate opportunity and circumstances for sleep, 3. and results in some form of daytime impairment" [1] (p19). For a diagnosis of insomnia, *all 3 criteria* must be met as noted in Box 1. Signs and symptoms of daytime impairment include fatigue, decreased mood or irritability, general malaise, cognitive impairments, and physical symptoms (headache, muscle tension, heart palpitations) [1]. For patients whose schedules do not allow 7–8 hours per night of uninterrupted sleep, or for those who wake up rested despite less than 7–8 hours of sleep, the diagnosis is not insomnia.

Chronic/acute/other insomnia

Insomnia has long been thought to be a disorder of hyperarousal. It is currently categorized as: (1) chronic (persisting >90 days and occurring at least 3 times per week), (2) acute (persisting <90 days and occurring at least 3 times per week), or (3) other [1]. As outlined in Table 2, subtypes of chronic insomnia exist, but are not stand-alone diagnoses, and the treatment does not change. Although most patients experience difficulty sleeping from time to time, a major concern with not addressing acute insomnia is that it could develop into chronic insomnia, which can trigger a depression [1]. According to the American Academy of Sleep Medicine (AASM), cognitive behavioral therapy for insomnia (CBTi) is the treatment for all insomnias, having a superior treatment record with longer-term recovery rates than hypnotic use alone [3].

Insomnia does not occur over one bad night of sleep, and it will not get better in one night; it will take time to "retrain the brain" to sleeping well. Clinicians and patients must be patient. For patients who do not meet the 3 criteria for diagnosis of insomnia, reassurance and education of sleep hygiene will

---

Box 1: Three criteria for insomnia

1. Persistent sleep difficulty with:
   - Sleep initiation (falling asleep within 20–30 minutes)
   - Duration (sleeping enough to feel rested)
   - Consolidation (staying asleep for ≥85% of time in bed)
   - Quality (good, satisfying sleep)
2. Inadequate opportunity and circumstances for sleep (7–8 hours)
3. Some form of daytime impairment (fatigue, general malaise, cognitive impairment, physical symptoms)

Data from American Academy of Sleep Medicine. International Classification of Sleep Disorders Third Edition. 2014. Darien, IL: American Academy of Sleep Medicine. ISBN: 0991543416.

Table 2
The insomnias

Types of insomnia	Characteristics
1. Chronic insomnia disorder	Occurs ≥3 times per week, has been present for ≥3 mo, takes ≥20–30 min to fall asleep or return to sleep, awakening ≥30 min before alarm/desired time
Subtypes of chronic insomnia	
Psychophysiologic	Patients with heightened arousal who worry about sleep, but who sleep well when not at home
Idiopathic	Patient who most likely experience "life-long" insomnia; may be genetic
Paradoxic	Patients who sleep better than perceived (adequate sleep per polysomnogram and electroencephalogram without next-day impairment)
Inadequate sleep hygiene	Patients who do not fix a set sleep/wake schedule and plan for 7–8 h of sleep/night (students studying for finals; mothers with newborns, and so forth)
Behavioral insomnia of childhood	Improper sleep training
Insomnia due to a mental disorder	Patients with bipolar disorder
Insomnia due to a medical condition	Patients with chronic pain, sleep-related breathing disorders, and so forth
Insomnia due to a drug or substance	Patients who abuse substances or are takings medications with alerting effects
2. Acute insomnia disorder	Occurs <3 times per week, has been present for <3 mo, takes ≥20–30 min to fall asleep or return to sleep, awakening ≥30 min before alarm/desired time; typically has a situational precipitating factor (death in family; relocation; illness; newborn)
3. Other insomnia disorder	
Excessive time in bed	Typically, a childhood behavior that includes being put to bed but not falling asleep
Short sleeper	Sleeps ≤6 h per night without next-day impairment; may be genetic

Data from American Academy of Sleep Medicine. International Classification of Sleep Disorders Third Edition. 2014. Darien, IL: American Academy of Sleep Medicine. ISBN: 0991543416.

probably be sufficient. For the patient whose work and life schedule does not permit for 7 to 8 hours of uninterrupted sleep per night, a lifestyle change may be necessary. Management of shift work schedules and circadian misalignment is beyond the scope of this article, but resources are available searching PubMed.

Diagnosis of insomnia
Insomnia is a clinical diagnosis as there are no imaging or laboratory studies that will confirm its presence. To confirm a diagnosis, the patient must meet all 3 criteria for insomnia *and* have at least 7 to 8 hours every night to dedicate to uninterrupted sleep.

According to the AASM [1], the following should be included in a thorough medical history:

- Past medical history: are there any comorbidities that affect sleep, such as chronic pain?
- Medications: are there any prescription, over-the-counter, or supplements that have an alerting effect? (See "Medications That Can Cause Insomnia" at https://www.nationaljewish.org/conditions/insomnia/causes/medicines-that-can-cause-insomnia)?
- Social history: what is the use of alcohol and tobacco? Is there exercise close to bedtime?
- Sleep history: what is the sleep environment like? (good mattress, cool room, quiet, dark, no TV), see Fig. 1

Easy to use, self-administered questionnaires can help both the clinician and patient determine the severity of insomnia and the presence of depression and anxiety. These include the Two-Week Sleep Diary that gives a powerful visual overview of sleep and wake throughout the night, the Insomnia Severity Scale (ISI) with 7 questions to achieve a probability score of insomnia, and the Patient Questionnaire Survey-9 (PHQ-9), which assists with screening for depression and anxiety.

Two-Week Sleep Diary
The Two-Week Sleep Diary may be the single most informational tool available to help clinician and patient identify patterns of good and poor sleep. Over a 2-week period, the patient blackens out boxes when asleep. An example of a Sleep Diary can be seen at http://yoursleep.aasmnet.org/pdf/sleepdiary.pdf.

Insomnia severity index
The ISI is a 7-question reliable and validated tool for assessment of insomnia severity. Internal consistency was measured as 0.74 using the Cronbach alpha coefficient [13] (for the "ISI", see: myhealth.va.gov/mhv-portal-web/insomnia-severity-index).

Patient Questionnaire Survey-9
The PHQ-9 screens severity of depression. Internal consistency was measured as 0.87 using the Cronbach alpha coefficient with good sensitivity (.83) and specificity (.72) [14] (for the "Patient Health Questionnaire-9," see www.bmedreport.com/archives/14638).

COMORBIDITES AND INSOMNIA

There are many health conditions associated with insomnia and most are familiar to the primary care clinician. Treating a complaint of insomnia should first address triggering health issues, such as chronic pain, depression, anxiety, menopause, and pregnancy, to name a few. Second, other sleep disorders, such as an irregular sleep-wake schedule, sleep apnea, or restless legs syndrome (RLS) can also be common causes of poor sleep. Any comorbid health condition or sleep disorder must be treated in conjunction with management of the insomnia complaint.

Identifying factors that may be contributing to insomnia symptoms is critical for the primary care clinician. *Acute insomnia* is often caused from an identifiable stressor, such as illness, death in the family, financial crisis, job-related stress, divorce, or relationship issues. *Chronic insomnia* is often associated with long-standing medical comorbidities, anxiety, depression, or posttraumatic stress disorder. Both acute and chronic pain are commonly cited as a sleep disruptors by patients complaining of insomnia. Menopause, with night sweats and hot flashes often includes sleep disturbance as a symptom. Although it is important to address these issues directly, many studies have found that CBTi can be an effective treatment tool for patients with insomnia and comorbid mood disorder, chronic pain, and menopausal sleep disturbance [15–18]. Both the use of, and withdrawal from, certain medications and substances also contributes to difficulty sleeping. A careful history of medication use and its discontinuation should be taken, with the inclusion of over-the-counter medications, herbal supplements, stimulants, and illicit drugs [1].

Sleep disordered breathing

Sleep disordered breathing (SDB) is a broad term, which encompasses several diagnoses, including obstructive sleep apnea (OSA), central or complex sleep apnea, and upper airway resistance syndrome (UARS). Of these, the most commonly seen are OSA and UARS [1]. Any evaluation of insomnia should include questions evaluating the risk of SDB. Undiagnosed and untreated SDB is present in 68%–80% of individuals with chronic insomnia, but is often overlooked as a possible etiology during the evaluation [19,20]. SDB is defined as any abnormalities in respirations during sleep. These are commonly grouped into (1) obstructive or (2) central apnea disorders. Some patients, however, may have components of both types of sleep apnea [1].

Obstructive sleep apnea

OSA is caused by either a full closing or narrowing of the upper airway resulting in desaturation during sleep [1]. It is the most common form of sleep apnea, with an estimated prevalence of 9% to 38% in the general population [21]. The incidence of OSA increases with age, after menopause in women, with an increased body mass index, and in those with a very narrow oropharynx. In some elderly groups, the prevalence has been reported as high as 90% in men and 78% in women [21]. Two powerful signs and symptoms of OSA include snoring during sleep (complaints usually coming from the bed partner) and excessive daytime sleepiness [22]. Complaints of either should clue the clinician to ask further questions.

Central apnea

Central apnea is characterized by an absent or reduced respiratory effort. Patients with central apnea may have a Cheyne-Stokes breathing pattern during sleep, most commonly seen in individuals with congestive heart failure and a reduced ejection fraction [1,23]. Central apnea is also seen in patients using opioids. This is a more complex form of sleep apnea to treat and suspicion of, or findings of, should trigger a referral to a sleep medicine specialist.

Evaluation for sleep disordered breathing

Evaluating for SDB is a critical component of an insomnia workup. Several validated clinical tools are available to screen for SDB. These tools include the STOP-BANG questionnaire for OSA (see questionnaire at: www.stop-bang.ca/) and the Epworth Sleepiness Scale (ESS) for excessive daytime sleepiness (see scale at: www.sleepapnea.org/wp-content/uploads/2017/02/ESS-PDF-1990-97.pdf) [24,25]. Patients with OSA are often so tired during the day they fall asleep at work, or when stopped at a red light. A score of ≥ 8 or 9 on the ESS would be concerning. Clinicians can also evaluate risk using the common signs and symptoms of sleep apnea, listed in Table 3. These include, but are not limited to difficulty with sleep initiation or maintenance, waking early and being unable to fall back asleep, loud snoring, nonrestorative sleep despite adequate hours of sleep, headache on waking, frequent nocturia, observed pauses in breathing during sleep, waking choking or gasping, excessive daytime sleepiness, fatigue, memory and cognition difficulties, daily napping, and drowsy or inattentive driving.

Any patient presenting with chronic insomnia who also has signs or symptoms of SDB should be evaluated with either a polysomnogram or a home sleep study. In some primary care settings, this can occur through referral to a local sleep medicine specialist or by direct ordering of either an in-lab polysomnogram or home sleep apnea testing. In more rural areas, a specialist may not be readily available. If this is the case, home sleep apnea testing can

Table 3
Signs and symptoms of sleep disordered breathing

Signs and clinical features	Symptoms
• Snoring	• Waking headache
• Observed pauses in breathing	• Insomnia
• Wakes gasping or choking	• Excessive daytime sleepiness
• Body mass index >35	• Nonrestorative sleep
• Neck circumference >16" in women, >17" in men	• Fatigue
• Mallampatti score of 3 or 4, crowded oropharynx with tongue scalloping and high arched palate	• Nocturia
	• Memory/concentration difficulty
• Diagnosis of: HTN, CAD, A fib, type 2 DM, CHF, mood disorder, or cognitive dysfunction, PCOS, hypothyroid, GERD	• Nocturnal GERD
	• Waking with dry mouth/ sore throat

Abbreviations: A fib, atrial fibrillation; CAD, coronary artery disease; CHF, congestive heart failure; GERD, gastroesophageal reflux disease; HTN, hypertension; PCOS, polycystic ovary syndrome; type 2 DM, type 2 diabetes mellitus.

Data from American Academy of Sleep Medicine. International Classification of Sleep Disorders Third Edition. 2014. Darien, IL: American Academy of Sleep Medicine. ISBN: 0991543416.

be ordered through online resources or a local durable medical equipment company. Home sleep apnea testing can underestimate the severity of SDB, but is more readily accessible and acceptable for many primary care situations [26]. Insurance coverage may also mandate an in-lab or home sleep testing study.

An apnea hypopnea is the number of times per hour a patient has reduced breathing or no breathing with a concomitant oxygen desaturation. A sleep study with an Apnea Hypopnea Index (AHI) of greater than 5 events per hour in a symptomatic patient should be treated with either continuous positive airway pressure (CPAP) or an oral mandibular advancement device. A patient with an AHI greater than 15 events per hour should be treated, even if they are asymptomatic [1,27]. Individuals with straight forward OSA, without significant sleep-related hypoxia, can often be managed in the primary care setting using autotitrating CPAP therapy [28].

If the patient shows signs of central or complex sleep apnea, they should be referred to a sleep disorder specialist for management. These patients are not appropriate for autotitrating CPAP, as this can increase the prevalence of central sleep apneas. Individuals with severe sleep apnea or sleep-related hypoxia should be referred to a sleep disorder specialist for a therapeutic polysomnogram study and management.

Restless legs syndrome

RLS is sensori-motor disorder characterized by a distinct circadian rhythm and thought to be caused by dopamine dysfunction and low iron stores. Often unexplainable and unpleasant sensations typically begin in the lower legs and, over time, extend to other parts of the body. The sensations begin in the late afternoon or early evening, worsen during the night time hours, and abate in the morning, following the circadian pattern of dopamine and iron nadirs in the brain [29] (Box 2). RLS adversely affects nighttime sleep due to the unpleasant sensations, but the treatment is different than for insomnia. RLS is a clinical diagnosis, for which the URGE mnemonic was created. All 4 criteria must be met for the diagnosis of RLS. As iron and dopamine production are closely tied, a ferritin level less than 75 ng/mL, in a patient who meets criteria for RLS, reveals inadequate iron stores. Iron repletion is recommended with an over-the-counter hematinic if the patient is symptomatic, or an iron

---

Box 2: Symptoms of restless legs syndrome
- Unusual sensations (urges) that typically begin in lower extremities
- Sensations (urges) begin in the late afternoon or early evening
- Sensations (urges) lessen or disappear in the morning and during the day (circadian presentation)
- Sensations (urges) are worse at rest
- Sensations (urges) immediately abate with movement

transfusion can be considered [29]. Consultation with a sleep disorder specialist should be considered for an iron transfusion (RLS). The clinician and patient can decide the benefits and risks of a low-dose dopaminergic to manage RLS symptoms [29]. Additional information can be found through the RLS Foundation at www.rls.org.

MANAGEMENT OF INSOMNIA

Treatment goals for insomnia include: (1) improvement in the quality of sleep and (2) lessening of daytime impairment/s [1]. The proven and "standard" treatment is CBTi, endorsed by the AASM and Behavioral Sleep Medicine [3,30]. In order of strength for treating insomnia, the 5 components of CBTi include: (1) sleep restriction therapy (SRT), (2) cognitive reconditioning, (3) stimulus control, (4) relaxation, and (5) sleep hygiene. One does not need to be a licensed therapist to offer CBTi to patients, it can be delivered in the primary health care setting [31]. CBTi can be delivered in different formats including face-to-face, in a group, and over the Internet.

Behavior is learned, and this includes poor sleep habits. CBTi functions with the understanding that behaviors can be modified and healthier ones learned. The goal is to "retrain the brain." The 5 components of CBTi that help lead to healthier sleep should be individualized for the patient, as each person's experience of sleep will be different and unique.

Components of cognitive behavioral therapy for insomnia

The homeostatic sleep drive is the single most important force to fall asleep and stay asleep [32]. For every 2 hours of wakefulness, most adult humans will require 1 hour of sleep; for 16 hours of wakefulness, 8 hours of sleep is required. When the sleep drive/debt is strong enough, there is little difficulty falling asleep and staying asleep. When a patient tries to sleep without sufficient sleep drive/debt, they will not sleep well. For example, if a patient goes to bed too early with the goal of "getting enough sleep for the next day" and is not tired, they will have difficulty falling asleep. To increase sleep debt/drive, the most effective therapy for insomnia is sleep restriction therapy (SRT). Early morning sunlight to set the body's internal clock, the circadian rhythm, for the day is essential.

Sleep restriction therapy

SRT does not limit the number of hours a patient is asleep, but it does limit the number of hours a patient is in bed tossing and turning. A Two-Week Sleep Diary is helpful to visualize and calculate the total number of hours a patient is in bed both lying awake and actually sleeping. A phone application may be useful. From the visual, clinician and patient can calculate actual time asleep. The goal is to limit time in bed to time asleep; this helps increase the sleep drive/debt. SRT instructions include:

1. Calculate the number of hours *actually asleep* per night (do not include tossing and turning) from a Two-Week Sleep Diary

2. Set a wake time for the next 2 weeks and commit to getting up, even if off work
3. Count backwards from the designated wake time the total number of hours actually asleep and add 30 minutes
   - Example: Designated wake time is 6 AM and actual asleep time is 6 hours/night—go to bed at 11:30 PM and get out of bed at 6 AM (do not forget to add the extra 30 minutes!)
4. Do not restrict sleep time to less than 5-1/2 to 6 hours/night, it might be unsafe to drive
5. Go to bed at the same time every night and get out of bed at the designated wake time for 2 weeks; do not nap during the day and do not go to bed earlier than set sleep time
   5a. At the end of week 1, if you are asleep 85% of your "sleep time," add 15 minutes to sleep, or, go to bed at 1115 PM
   5b. At the end of week 1, if you are sleeping less than 85% of your "sleep time," subtract 15 minutes, or go to bed at 11:45 PM
6. Repeat steps 3–5a. and 5b [18]

Cognitive therapy
Cognitive therapy is examining, challenging, and reforming dysfunctional beliefs about sleep with a therapist or by self-examination using a diary [33]. The latter includes requesting patients to write down ruminating thoughts that keep them awake during the night and examine them in the morning. Before sleep time, patients should make lists of all that needs to be done the next day. This helps change the mantra from "I cannot sleep" to "I will relearn to sleep well."

Stimulus control
Stimulus control helps to "retrain the brain" by association. The bed should only be for sex and sleep. The bed should not be for eating, drinking, watching TV, and so forth, as these are activities associated with alertness and wakefulness. Stimulus control includes setting a sleep and wake time and sticking to it every day, even on vacations and holidays, and includes no napping. To strengthen the association of bed = sleep, if the patient is not asleep within 20 to 30 minutes after going to bed, they should get up out of bed and engage in a boring activity, in dim light. When sleepy, the patient may return to bed. If the patient is again not asleep within 20 to 30 minutes, they should get out of bed. Over one to two nights, this will increase sleep drive/debt.

Relaxation
Relaxation is learning to let go of tension through progressive muscle relaxation or mindfulness. This is helpful for most patients in multiple situations.

Sleep hygiene
Sleep hygiene is good common sense about the sleep environment: keep the room dark and cool, go to bed and wake up at the same time every day, do not take stimulants close to sleep time (caffeine). The key is to take each recommendation and individualize it with the patient. A good question for the

clinician to use is, "How do you see yourself creating a good sleep environment?" See Box 3 (https://www.sleepfoundation.org/articles/sleep-hygiene).

Modalities to deliver cognitive behavioral therapy for insomnia

CBTi can be delivered as face-to-face counseling with a trained therapist, to a self-paced schedule via the Internet. Delivery will largely depend on clinician resources and patient needs.

- CBTi includes 4 to 8 two-hour one-on-one counseling sessions with a therapist
- Brief behavioral therapy for insomnia includes 2 to 4 two-hour one-on-one counseling sessions, it could also include a single 45-minute session with a 30-minute "booster" appointment and might include telephone follow-up
- Abbreviated cognitive behavioral therapy includes 2, 25-minute sessions with a therapist and a booklet
- One-shot behavioral therapy for Insomnia targets the 2 most powerful components of CBTi: (1) SRT and (2) cognitive therapy and is appropriate for the primary care setting. The clinician can have booklets premade for patients with what the authors call the "Already Ready Booklet." A follow-up appointment in 2 weeks, billed as a health behavior visit, could be considered [33] (Box 4)
- Group delivered one-shot behavioral therapy [34,35]
  ○ One-shot behavioral therapy uses the 3Ds: *D*etect sleep habits using a diary (could use a phone application), *D*etach from poor sleep habits with stimulus control, and *D*istract with cognitive imaging and relaxation [35]
- Internet-based CBTi is online and patient self-paced. A systematic review and meta-analysis revealed no statistically significant differences between Internet-based and therapist-assisted CBTi when examining patient ISI scores, total sleep time (want 7–8 hours), and sleep efficiency (time in bed actually asleep; want ≥85%) [36] (Box 5)

Box 3: Sleep hygiene recommendations

- If you do nap, limit to 15–30 minutes
- Avoid stimulants before sleep time (tobacco, caffeine)
- Exercise daily to promote a sense of well-being, but not close to bedtime
- Avoid stomach upsetting food before sleep time
- Set a sleep time and a wake time and stick to it
- Get bright light (preferably sun) first thing in the morning
- Use dim light in the late afternoon and evening (stay away from cell phones and lap tops in the evening, and especially in bed)
- Create a pleasant sleep environment: cool room, dark room, no distractions, good mattress, clean linen (especially pillow case for sense of smell), ear plugs, white noise machine

Data from Sleep Hygiene. National Foundation for Sleep. Available at: https://www.sleepfoundation.org/articles/sleep-hygiene.

Box 4: The "already ready" folder

- Two-Week Sleep Diary, see http://yoursleep.aasmnet.org/pdf/sleepdiary.pdf
- ISI, see: myhealth.va.gov/mhv-portal-web/insomnia-severity-index
- PHQ-9, see: www.bmedreport.com/archives/14638
- STOP-BANG Questionnaire, www.stopbang.ca
- ESS, www.sleepapnea.org/wp-content/uploads/2017/02/ESS-PDF-1990-97.pdf
- URGE mnemonic for RLS (see section "Restless legs syndrome")
- How to calculate for SRT (see section "Sleep restriction theraphy")
- Sleep hygiene recommendations, see https://www.sleepfoundation.org/articles/sleep-hygiene
- Online patient resources, see http://www.sleepreviewmag.com/2014/12/online-options-insomnia-therapy/; https://mobile.va.gov/app/cbt-i-coach
- Books resources:
  - Carney & Manber. 2013. Goodnight mind. Turn off your noisy thoughts & get a good night's sleep.
  - Carney & Manber. 2009. Quiet your mind and get to sleep: Solutions to insomnia for those with depression, anxiety or chronic pain.

PHARMACOLOGIC TREATMENT

After comorbidities have been addressed and treated (eg, chronic insomnia, OSA) pharmacologic treatment of *chronic insomnia* may be necessary *on a short-term basis*. In addition, not all patients have access to CBTi and CBTi is not completely effective for all patients with insomnia symptoms. When medication is necessary, *sleep onset* versus *sleep maintenance* insomnia must be considered; the former being difficulty falling asleep and the latter difficulty staying asleep.

To assist clinicians, an AASM task force was convened to examine commonly used medications and supplements for the treatment of chronic insomnia [2,37]. Applying the Grading of Recommendations Assessment, Development, and Evaluation to randomized controlled trials gathered

Box 5: Internet CBT-I resources for patients

Phone app

- https://mobile.va.gov/app/cbt-i-coach

Online

- http://www.sleepreviewmag.com/2014/12/online-options-insomnia-therapy/ (CBTforInsomnia; CBT-I Coach; Shuti; Sleepio; RESTORE; SLEEPTUTOR)
- www.myshuti.com
- https://www.cbtforinsomnia.com/

during a systematic review, medication recommendations were made. A recommendation of STRONG is the preferred treatment under most circumstances. A recommendation of WEAK has less evidence of effectiveness, but on an individual basis, may be effective for that patient. Box 6 is adapted from the task force summary and all recommendations are rated as WEAK [2,37].

Box 6: Pharmacology for insomnia – all recommendations WEAK

Sleep onset insomnia – Difficulty falling asleep
  Sonata (zoleplon) – non-BNZ hypnotic
  Ambien (zolpidem) – non-BNZ hypnotic
  Halcion (triazolam) – BNZ
  Restoril (temazepam) – BNZ
  Rozerem (ramelteon) – melatonin receptor agonist
Recommend do NOT use for sleep onset
  Gabitril (tiagabine) – GABA reuptake inhibitor
  Desyrel (trazodone) – sedating SSRI
  Benadryl (diphenhydramine) – antihistamine
  Melatonin – hormone
  Tryptophan – amino acid
  Valerian – plant root
Sleep maintenance insomnia – Difficulty staying asleep
  Belsomra (survorexant) – selective, dual orexin receptor antagonist
  Lunesta (eszopiclone) – non-BNZ hypnotic
  Ambien (zolpidem) – non-BNZ hypnotic
  Restoril (temazepam) – BNZ
Recommend do NOT use for sleep maintenance
  Gabitril (tiagabine) – GABA reuptake inhibitor
  Desyrel (trazodone) sedating SSRI
  Sinequan (doxepin) TCA
  Benadryl (diphenhydramine) – antihistamine
  Melatonin – hormone
  Tryptophan – amino acid
  Valerian – plant root

Abbreviations: BNZ, benzodiazepine; GABA, gamma-amino butyric acid; SSRI, serotonin reuptake inhibitor; TCA, tricyclic antidepressant.
Data from Sateia MJ, Buysse DJ, Krystal AD et al. Clinical practice guideline for the pharmacologic treatment of chronic insomnia in adults: an American Academy of Sleep Medicine clinical practice guideline. *J Clin Sleep Med.* 2017;13(2):307–349; and Schutte-Rodin S, Broch L, Buysse D, Dorsey C, et al. Clinical Guideline for the evaluation and management of chronic insomnia in adults. J Clin Sleep Med 2008; 4(5):487-504.

A Cochrane review of eszopiclone use for insomnia revealed its usefulness for sleep onset and sleep maintenance insomnia. Over the short term (4 weeks), medium term (4–24 weeks), and long term (longer than 6 months) sleep efficacy was better for eszopiclone when compared with placebo in the review which included 14 studies (N = 4732). Overall, use of eszopiclone resulted in a 12-minute decrease of falling sleep (mean difference [MD] = −11.94 min; 95% CI, −16.03 to − 7.86), a 17-minute decrease of waking up after falling asleep (MD = −17.02 min; 95% CI, −24.89 to −9.15), and a 28-minute increase in total time asleep (MD = 27.70 min; 95% CI, 20.30–35.09) (x p2).

However, there were more adverse events with eszopiclone compared with placebo: unpleasant taste (risk difference [RD] = 0.18; 95% CI, 0.14–0.21), dry mouth (RD = 0.04; 95% CI, 0.02–0.06), somnolence (RD = 0.04; 95% CI, 0.02–0.06), and dizziness (RD = 0.03; 95% CI, 0.01–0.05) [38] (p2).

The authors' conclusion was that "eszopiclone appears to be an efficient drug with moderate effects on sleep onset and maintenance. There was no or little evidence of harm *if taken as recommended*." When prescribing hypnotics, the following suggestions may be helpful:

- Use only when necessary
- Avoid concomitant use of alcohol
- Start with lowest dose and titrate upward slowly ("low and slow")
- Titrate dose down when sleeping better
- Use for the shortest period possible
- Use lower doses for elderly
- Use with extreme caution during pregnancy
- Use short-acting non-benzodiazepine (non-BNZ) for sleep onset
- Use BNZ with longer half-life for sleep maintenance
- Use sedating antidepressant over hypnotic if comorbid depression/anxiety
- Avoid BNZ if comorbid SDB such as OSA
- Plan for a full 6 hours, preferably 8 hours, of dedicated sleep time
- If medication adversely affects daytime activities, stop medication and call clinician

Treatment of *acute insomnia* is usually time limited, resolving with the stressor event. For instance, a new mother will eventually get better sleep once a breast-feeding pattern is established with her newborn. Family discord or employment upsets eventually resolve. Whether or not to supplement short term with a short-acting non-BNZ would be between the clinician and patient. Depression and anxiety might require treatment by a professional.

WHEN TO REFER

Sleep disorders can be very complex and beyond the time allowed in a primary care clinic to treat and manage properly. The AASM recommends patients be referred if history and/or treatments meet the following [1]:

- Signs and symptoms of OSA
- Symptoms of RLS/periodic leg movement disorder

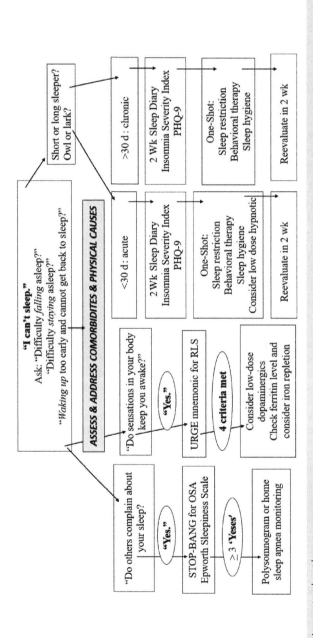

Fig. 2. Insomnia algorithm.

- Use of daily sedative-hypnotics for ≥30 days
- Chronic insomnia not responsive to cognitive behavioral therapy
- Patients with comorbidities

PHONE APPS

Phone applications that record sleep may be helpful [39] in detecting poor habits and transferred onto the Two-Week Sleep Diary for good visual accounting. It could be helpful for patients to follow improvement in sleep consolidation with SRT. However, phone applications are not a substitute for polysomnography or home sleep testing for diagnosis of OSA or other sleep disorders that require multiple recordings, such as AHI, electroencephalogram, electrocardiogram, SaO_2 [40].

SUMMARY

Time constraints in the primary care setting often preclude ongoing visits for CBTi. Nonetheless, the primary care clinician could have ready access to the STOP-BANG and ESS questionnaires to screen for OSA. An Already Ready Booklet that includes the ISI, the PHQ-9, a Two-Week Sleep Diary, Sleep Hygiene Recommendations, and information on Sleep Restriction could be handy. A list of resources would allow the patient to consider Internet-based CBTi. If managed in the primary care clinic, the patient should return in 2 weeks with the Sleep Diary to go over where improvements can be made. The authors hope an algorithm may be useful during a busy clinic day (Fig. 2).

References

[1] American Academy of Sleep Medicine. International classification of sleep disorders. 3rd edition. Darien (IL): American Academy of Sleep Medicine; 2014.

[2] Schutte-Rodin S, Broch L, Buysse D, et al. Clinical guideline for the evaluation and management of chronic insomnia in adults. J Clin Sleep Med 2008;4(5):487–504.

[3] American Academy of Sleep Medicine. Practice parameters for the psychological and behavioral treatment of insomnia in: guidelines at-a-glance. A resource by the American Academy of Sleep Medicine. Darien (IL): AASM; 2018.

[4] Ohayon MM. Epidemiology of insomnia: what we know and what we still need to learn. Sleep Med Rev 2002;6:97–111, 2.

[5] Kyle SD, Morgan K, Espie CA. Insomnia and health-related quality of life. Sleep Med Rev 2010;14:69–82.

[6] Institute of Medicine. Sleep disorders and sleep deprivation: an unmet public health problem. Washington, DC: The National Academies Press; 2006.

[7] Zielinski MR, McKenna JT. Functions and mechanisms of sleep. AIMS Neurosci 2016;3(1): 67–104.

[8] Liu Y, Wheaton AG, Chapman DP, et al. Prevalence of healthy sleep duration among adults — United States, 2014. MMWR Morb Mortal Wkly Rep 2016;65:137–41.

[9] Watson NF, Badr MS, Belenky G, et al. Recommended amount of sleep for a healthy adult: a joint consensus statement of the American Academy of Sleep Medicine and Sleep Research Society. J Clin Sleep Med 2015;11(6):591–2.

[10] Gallicchio L, Kalesa B. Sleep duration and mortality: a systematic review and meta-analysis. J Sleep Res 2008;18:148–58.

[11] Shi G, Xing L, Wu D, et al. A rare mutation of β1-adrenergic receptor affects sleep/wake behaviors. Neuron 2019;103(6):1044–55.e7.

[12] Buysse DJ. Sleep health: can we define it? Does it matter? Sleep 2014;37(1):9–17.

[13] Bastien CH, Vallières A, Morin CM. Validation of the Insomnia Severity Index as an outcome measure for insomnia research. Sleep Med 2001;2(4):297–307.

[14] Beard C, Hsu KJ, Rifkin LS, et al. Validation of the PHQ-9 in a psychiatric sample. J Affect Disord 2016;193:267–73.

[15] Guthrie KA, Larson JC, Ensrud KE, et al. Effects of pharmacologic and nonpharmacologic interventions on insomnia symptoms and self-reported sleep quality in women with hot flashes: a pooled analysis of individual participant data from four MsFLASH trials. Sleep 2018;41(1); https://doi.org/10.1093/sleep/zsx190.

[16] Koffel E, Amundson A, Wisdom JP. Exploring the meaning of cognitive behavioral therapy for insomnia for patients with chronic pain. Pain Med 2019;pnz144; https://doi.org/10.1093/pm/pnz144.

[17] Drake CL, Kalmbach DA, Todd J, et al. Treating chronic insomnia in postmenopausal women: a randomized clinical trial comparing cognitive-behavioral therapy for insomnia, sleep restriction therapy, and sleep hygiene education. Sleep 2019;42(2):zsy21.

[18] Kalmbach DA, Cheng P, Arnedt JT, et al. Improving daytime functioning, work performance, and quality of life in postmenopausal women with insomnia: comparing cognitive behavioral therapy for insomnia, sleep restriction therapy, and sleep hygiene education. J Clin Sleep Med 2019;15(7):999–1010.

[19] Krakow B, McIver ND, Ulibarri VA, et al. Prospective randomized controlled trial on the efficacy of continuous positive airway pressure and adaptive servo-ventilation in the treatmen of chronic complex insomnia. EClinicalMedicine 2019;13:57–73.

[20] Luyster FS, Buysse DJ, Strollo PJ Jr. Comorbid insomnia and obstructive sleep apnea: challenges for clinical practice and research. J Clin Sleep Med 2010;6(2):196–204.

[21] Senaratna CV, Perret JL, Lodge C, et al. Prevalence of obstructive sleep apnea in the general population: a systematic review. Sleep Med Rev 2017;34:70–81.

[22] Stansbury RC, Strollo PJ. Clinical manifestations of sleep apnea. J Thorac Dis 2015;7(9):E298–310.

[23] Aurora RN, Chowdhuri S, Ramar K, et al. The treatment of central sleep apnea syndromes in adults: practice parameters with an evidence-based literature review and meta-analyses. SLEEP 2012;35(1):17–40.

[24] Epstein LJ, Kristo D, Strollo PJ, et al. Clinical guideline for the evaluation, management and long-term care of obstructive sleep apnea in adults. J Clin Sleep Med 2009;5(3):263–76.

[25] Nagappa M, Liao P, Wong J, et al. Validation of the STOP-Bang questionnaire as a screening tool for obstructive sleep apnea among different populations: a systematic review and meta-analysis. PLoS One 2015;10(12):e0143697.

[26] Andrade L, Paiva T. Ambulatory versus laboratory polysomnography in obstructive sleep apnea: comparative assessment of quality, clinical efficacy, treatment compliance, and quality of life. J Clin Sleep Med 2018;14(8):1323–31.

[27] Patil SP, Ayappa IA, Caples SM, et al. Treatment of adult obstructive sleep apnea with positive airway pressure: an American Academy of Sleep Medicine clinical practice guideline. J Clin Sleep Med 2019;15(2):335–43.

[28] Sánchez-Quiroga MÁ, Corral J, Gómez-de-Terreros FJ, et al. Primary care physicians can comprehensively manage sleep apnea patients: a non-inferiority randomized controlled rial. Am J Respir Crit Care Med 2018; https://doi.org/10.1164/rccm.201710-2061OC.

[29] Aurora RN, Kristo DA, Bista SR, et al. Update to the AASM clinical practice guideline: "the treatment of restless legs syndrome and periodic limb movement disorder in adults—an update for 2012: practice parameters with an evidence-based systematic review and meta-analyses. Sleep 2012;35(8):1037.

[30] Morgenthaler T, Kramer M, Alessi C, et al. Practice parameters for the psychological and behavioral treatment of insomnia: an update. An American academy of sleep medicine report. Sleep 2006;29(11):1415–9.

[31] Dorlinger LM, Fortin AH, Foran-Tuller KA. Training primary care physicians in cognitive behavioral therapy: a review of the literature. Patient Educ Couns 2016;99:1285–92.

[32] Muto V, Jaspar M, Meyer C, et al. Local modulation of human brain responses by circadian rhythmicity and sleep debt. Science 2016;353(6300):687–90.

[33] Ellis J. Cognitive behavioral therapy for insomnia and acute insomnia. Sleep Med Clin 2019;14:267–74.

[34] Boulin P, Ellwood C, Ellis JG. Group vs. individual treatment for acute insomnia: a pilot study evaluating a "one-shot" treatment. Brain Sci 2017;7(1):1.

[35] Ellis JG, Cushing T, Germain A. Treating acute insomnia: a randomized controlled trial of a "single-shot" of cognitive behavioral therapy for insomnia. Sleep 2015;38(6):971–8.

[36] Seyffert M, Lagisetty P, Landgraf J, et al. Internet delivered cognitive behavioral therapy to treat insomnia: a systematic review and meta-analysis. PLoS One 2016;11(2):e0149139.

[37] Sateia MJ, Buysse DJ, Krystal AD, et al. Clinical practice guideline for the pharmacologic treatment of chronic insomnia in adults: an American Academy of Sleep Medicine clinical practice guideline. J Clin Sleep Med 2017;13(2):307–49.

[38] Rösner S, Englbrecht C, Wehrle R, et al. Eszopiclone for insomnia. Cochrane Database Syst Rev 2018;(10):CD010703.

[39] Shin JC, Kim J, Grigsby-Toussaint D. Mobile phone interventions for sleep disorders and sleep quality: a systematic review. JMIR Mhealth Uhealth 2017;5(9):e131.

[40] Choi YK, Demiris G, Lin S-Y, et al. Smartphone applications to support sleep self-management: review and evaluation. J Clin Sleep Med 2018;14(10):1783–90.

Pediatrics

Advances in Family Practice Nursing 2 (2020) 145–157

ELSEVIER
MOSBY

ADVANCES IN FAMILY PRACTICE NURSING

Teens and Vaping
What You Need to Know

Check for
updates

Jeannie Rodriguez, PhD, RN, APRN*,
Debbie Silverstein, MSN, RN, FNP, Irene Yang, PhD, RN

Emory University Nell Hodgson Woodruff School of Nursing, 1520 Clifton Road, Northeast,
Atlanta, GA 30322, USA

Keywords
• Youth • ENDS • Electronic cigarettes

Key points
• Rapid growth in electronic nicotine delivery systems (ENDS) use since 2010 is particularly evident among youth.
• Much remains unknown about the impact of constituents emitted by e-cigarettes.
• Youth may be particularly vulnerable to nicotine exposure because of the structural and neurochemical development occurring in their central nervous system.
• In addition to screening for use and susceptibility to use, health care providers should also consider screening youth who already use ENDS for nicotine dependence.

INTRODUCTION

Electronic nicotine delivery systems (ENDS) [1], commonly known as e-cigarettes or vapes, are growing in popularity in the United States [2]. These devices vaporize liquids that typically contain nicotine, flavorings, and other additives [3], which are inhaled by the user. The US Surgeon General has called e-cigarette use among youth a public health concern and considers use by youth of any product containing nicotine, including e-cigarettes, unsafe [2].

Rapid growth in ENDS use since 2010 [4] is particularly evident among youth [3]. Between 2011 and 2018, current e-cigarette use among high school

Drs J. Rodriguez and I. Yang wish to acknowledge financial support by a pilot project grant from the Emory University HERCULES Center (P30 ES019776). Dr J. Rodriguez acknowledges financial support from NIEHS/EPA (P50ES026071) and NIDMH (R01 MD009746). Dr I. Yang acknowledges financial support from NINR (K01 NR016971-01A1) and (3P30NR018090-02S2).

*Corresponding author. E-mail address: Jeannie.rodriguez@emory.edu

https://doi.org/10.1016/j.yfpn.2020.01.010
2589-420X/20/

students increased from 1.5% to 20.8% [5,6], with those reporting ever using e-cigarettes as high as 37.7% [2]. A similar trend exists beyond the United States [3]. Middle school students are vaping as well. In 2018, prevalence of current e-cigarette use among middle school students was 4.9% [5], with 13.5% of middle school students reporting ever trying e-cigarettes [2]. Despite concerted tobacco prevention and control strategies like smoke-free policies that include e-cigarettes, and media campaigns warning about the risks of youth tobacco product use [5,7], vaping prevalence is increasing, and e-cigarettes are now the most commonly used form of nicotine among youth and young adults [5].

This health behavior among youth is particularly significant given the highly addictive properties of nicotine [2]. Those who initiate e-cigarette use during their youth will have a higher risk for life-long nicotine addiction and any subsequent health effects [2]. Developmental factors typically noted during adolescence, such as impulsivity, deficits in attention, and incomplete executive functioning, can compound the likelihood of risk-taking behaviors and subsequent addiction [2]. Little research has been conducted examining the short- and long-term health effects of e-cigarette use among youth, and scant guidance concerning screening and counseling is available for health professionals. The purpose of this article is to summarize what is known about e-cigarettes and their health effects on youth and provide health care professionals with some initial direction with regard to screening and counseling youth e-cigarette users and their families.

OVERVIEW OF E-CIGARETTES

E-cigarettes are alternative nicotine delivery devices that heat liquids, typically containing nicotine, flavorings, and other additives, into an inhalable aerosol. They may also be called, "e-cigs," "vapes," "vape pens," mods," and "tanks" [8]. These devices generally comprise a liquid, a heating element, and a battery [3].

E-cigarettes can generally be categorized as first-, second-, or third-generation devices [8]. First-generation devices are "closed systems" and are sometimes called "cigalikes" for their close resemblance to the conventional cigarette (Fig. 1) [9]. These devices are either disposable or reloadable with cartridges prefilled with e-liquid, or nicotine-containing solutions [9]. These closed systems are not customizable, meaning that vapers must either dispose of them or reload with brand-matched prefilled cartridges [9].

Second-generation devices tend to be larger, have a more powerful battery linked to an atomizer, and a refillable tank that the user can fill with their choice of e-liquid with different flavors and nicotine concentrations. Because of the ability of the user to open the device and customize them, this generation of devices is generally considered "open system" (Fig. 2). These devices also often look like a fountain pen and are frequently referred to as "vape-pens" [8,10].

Third-generation devices are even larger and may be called "mods" (Fig. 3) [8]. These devices are also considered "open system" and highly customizable

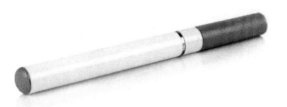

Fig. 1. First-generation "closed system" or "cigalike." (*From* Gmstockstudio/shuttershock.com.)

in terms of e-liquid, mouthpieces, and variable voltage options [9]. In general, open systems are capable of delivering higher levels of nicotine and are generally bulkier and heavier than closed systems [9]. This "open system" may also make these devices more susceptible to tampering with the addition of other chemicals, including tetrahydrocannabinol.

The most current generation of e-cigarettes represents a new category of products that are sleeker, with a high-tech design, easily rechargeable batteries, and high nicotine delivery [8]. These devices may also be called "pod mods" [11]. JUUL (Fig. 4), which emerged in 2016 and quickly established itself as a leading pod mod product by early 2018, has been followed by several similar products, like Suorin Drop and myblu.

The vaping epidemic

The explosion in the ENDS market has been accompanied by a dramatic increase in its use [12]. More than 15% of adults have used ENDS products, with the majority being between the ages of 18 and 44 [13]. The products are popular among conventional cigarette users [14], who may be drawn to the marketing of e-cigarettes as safer alternatives to conventional cigarettes, and the tobacco naive, or youth who have never smoked conventional cigarettes before initiating ENDS use [15].

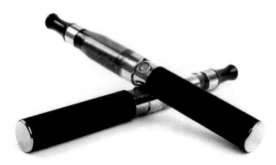

Fig. 2. Second-generation "open system" or "vape-pens." (*From* Gmstockstudio/shuttershock.com.)

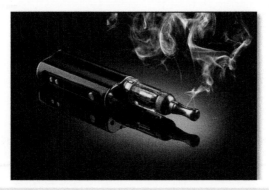

Fig. 3. Third-generation "open system" or "mod." (*From* Gresei/shuttershock.com.)

Popular products and their appeal for adolescents

Vapers have access to a US market of at least 466 brands and 7764 flavors of e-cigarettes [16,17]. JUUL is currently the top-selling e-cigarette brand in the United States [18]. In fact, the rapidly increasing prevalence of vaping among adolescents has paralleled the growing popularity of this brand [18]. News and social media sites report widespread "juuling" by students at school [19].

Youth report several reasons for starting to vape. These reasons include curiosity, the appeal of attractive-sounding flavors, peer influence [20,21], and the ability to easily conceal devices from authority figures [22]. Popular pod mod devices, like JUUL, have a sleek, modern design with customizable adhesive covers, or "skins," and are extremely easy to use [11]. Although many e-cigarette devices require purchase of solutions from independent manufacturers, manual refilling, and user calibration, youth can simply open their pod mod starter kit package, slide a flavor pod into their device, and start vaping [11].

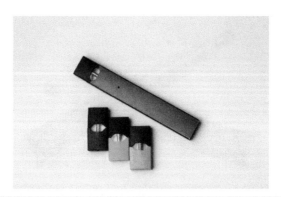

Fig. 4. "Pod mod" products like JUUL. (*From* Mary Caroline/shutterstock.com.)

Smoking cessation is not reported by youth as a reason for taking up vaping [23]. Despite the fact that one of the strongest predictors of e-cigarette use is conventional smoking, this is not the case in the adolescent population [24]. For example, in 2012, an estimated 160,000 students who had never used conventional cigarettes reported ever having vaped [25], making e-cigarette use among nicotine-naive adolescents a growing public health concern.

Current regulations relevant to adolescent use

In 2016, the US Food and Drug Administration's (FDA) Center for Tobacco Products finalized a rule to regulate e-cigarette products [26]. This ruling enables the FDA to establish product standards and regulate the manufacturing, importing, packaging, labeling, advertising, promotion, sale, and distribution of e-cigarettes, including components and parts of e-cigarettes [26]. The regulation set a deadline of August 8, 2022 in order to determine whether existing e-cigarette products can remain on the market [8], although the deadline for most flavored e-cigarettes has been moved up 1 year to August 8, 2021, addressing the products that are most likely to entice youth [27]. The regulation also established a federal minimum age of 18 for the sale of all tobacco products, including e-cigarettes [26], and several states and localities have established a minimum age of 21 for the sale of tobacco products [28]. Retailers must check the photo identification of everyone under the age of 27 who attempts to purchase e-cigarettes [8]. The FDA, however, has not yet implemented age verification regulations for online and other non–face-to-face purchases, creating an online environment whereby only a portion of Internet vendors provide age warnings or effective age verification [8]. Also included within this regulation is the prohibition of free samples of e-cigarettes and their components and vending machine sales of e-cigarettes (except in facilities restricted to adults over the age of 18) [8].

The rapid increase of vaping among youth attests to the ineffectiveness of these regulation efforts. In response to the latest adolescent e-cigarette use statistics, JUUL has stopped selling their e-liquid pods to retail stores, enhanced their online age-verification system, and report that they are working to remove inappropriate third-party social media content [18]. The FDA has initiated a "Youth Tobacco Prevention Plan" focused on preventing access, curbing marketing of e-cigarettes toward youth, and educating youth on the dangers of any tobacco product, including e-cigarettes [29].

HEALTH EFFECTS

Although evidence suggests that using e-cigarettes is substantially less harmful than inhaling smoke from conventional cigarettes, much remains unknown about the impact of particular constituents emitted by e-cigarettes. For example, flavors used in e-liquids have been approved by the FDA for consumption, but not for inhalation [24], and the impact of these flavoring chemicals as inhaled aerosols is unknown. This lack of knowledge combined with constant innovation in the e-cigarette industry emphasizes the urgent need for continued research and monitoring of the health impact, addictiveness, and toxicity of e-cigarettes [8].

Although some health benefits like reduced blood pressure exist for conventional smokers who switch to e-cigarettes, research on the impact of vaping for naive users is, as yet, inconclusive. There is some evidence, however, to suggest that vaping is not innocuous. Adverse event reports to the FDA from e-cigarette use include mouth and throat irritation, nausea, headache, and dry cough [3]. Moderate to strong evidence exists for increased cough and wheeze in adolescents who use e-cigarettes; an association between e-cigarette use and increased asthma exacerbations [30]; and increased heart rate resulting from nicotine exposure with e-cigarette use [3,30]. Further research is needed to demonstrate this impact and understand the underlying physiologic mechanism.

Other dangers related to e-cigarettes

There is conclusive evidence that e-cigarette devices can explode and cause burns and projectile injuries, dependent on battery quality, storage conditions, and device modifications by the user [30]. From 2012 to 2015, there were 92 reported e-cigarette–related events in the United States that resulted from over-heating/fire/explosion events [3]. Half of these caused injuries like thermal burns, lacerations, or smoke inhalation [3]. Beyond inhalation, other modes of exposure to e-liquids, such as ingestion, dermal contact, or injection, although rare, are dangerous, with effects including seizures, anoxic brain injury, vomiting, lactic acidosis, and even death [30,31]. More recently, there have been concerns about vaping and the development of an acute pulmonary illness. The Centers for Disease Control and Prevention issued a health advisory on August 30, 2019 concerning a multistate outbreak of a severe pulmonary disease associated with e-cigarette use [32].

Chemical components of e-cigarettes and vapor

Although e-cigarettes are marketed as safe products, at least 60 chemical compounds have been detected in e-liquids, with even more known to be inhaled as the liquids are aerosolized [30]. Although some of these compounds have not yet been identified, some are known to be harmful or potentially harmful.

Nicotine, e-cigarettes, and the teenage brain

Nicotine levels in e-cigarettes vary across manufacturers, e-liquid concentrations, devices, and individual puffing habits [3]. Nicotine delivered via conventional cigarette smoking is known to be powerfully addictive [33]. Some e-cigarette products, however, are able to deliver nicotine almost as efficiently as a conventional cigarette. For example, manufacturers of the JUUL product claim that a single JUUL cartridge is roughly equal to a pack of cigarettes, or 200 cigarette puffs, with delivery of nicotine up to 2.7 times faster than other e-cigarettes, increasing the potential for addiction and putting a new generation of youth at risk of nicotine dependence and future conventional cigarette use [8]. Even closed system e-cigarettes that deliver lower concentrations of nicotine to the user are not without risk [24]. These lower-yield devices may function as "starter products" designed to deliver low doses of nicotine without causing adverse effects, resulting in a cascade effect of increased tolerance, seeking products that deliver higher nicotine doses, and eventual dependence [24].

Youth may be particularly vulnerable to nicotine exposure because of the structural and neurochemical development occurring in their central nervous system [34]. Nicotine exposure from e-cigarettes affects neurotransmitter activity and increases the rewarding effects of other drugs of abuse [34]. Evidence supporting this relationship can be found in epidemiologic studies that show that the use of ENDS is correlated with the use of other tobacco products, marijuana, and alcohol [3]. Nicotine exposure to the adolescent brain may also contribute to attention and cognitive deficits and exacerbate mood disorders [34]. Overall, even low doses of nicotine put adolescent vapers at risk for long-term neurologic effects [24]. Given the speed and yield of nicotine delivery by products like JUUL, the risk to the developing adolescent brain is an important consideration.

Other chemical constituents
Various other, potentially toxic, compounds [35–41], some of which are created by the thermal breakdown of the ingredients in the e-liquid [24], have been identified in ENDS aerosols. These compounds include tobacco-specific nitrosamines, ultrafine particulate matter, polycyclic aromatic hydrocarbons, volatile organic compounds like benzene, carbonyls like formaldehyde and diacetyl, acrolein, and heavy metals like nickel, tin, and lead [2,3,42–44]. Although some studies suggest that these constituents are lower in e-cigarette aerosols compared with combustible cigarette smoke [3], levels are dependent on device differences. For example, increasing voltage increases the yield of formaldehyde, acetaldehyde, and acetone [45,46] within the range of that observed in tobacco smoke [45]. Recently, researchers have noted that flavorings added to e-cigarette liquids when mixed with other additives can become unstable and can form new compounds during storage and use [47]. These compounds are not reported as ingredients by manufacturers, making scientific investigation more challenging [47].

Research has also linked some of these constituents with adverse outcomes. For example, volatile organic compounds are associated with irritation, headaches, and organ damage; polycyclic aromatic hydrocarbons are known carcinogens [24]; and heavy metals and particulate matter have been associated with respiratory irritation and impaired lung function [48,49]. In vitro cellular studies have shown that the soluble components of e-cigarettes cause oxidative stress, inflammatory effects, DNA damage, mutagenesis, and decreased cell viability [30,50,51]. Certain flavors of e-cigarette liquid, like cinnamon, have also been found to be more cytotoxic than others [3]. These findings support the biological plausibility that long-term exposure to e-cigarette aerosols could potentially increase the risk of cancer [30].

Nicotine salts in e-liquids

Newer brands of e-cigarettes, like JUUL, contain nicotine salts in the e-liquid [8]. These nicotine salts allow pod mods, like JUUL, to deliver high concentrations of nicotine without the unpleasant experiences that corresponding doses of nicotine would elicit for conventional smokers. According to their advertisements, nicotine salt solutions contain nicotine concentrations up to 10 times higher than their e-cigarette counterparts that use free-base nicotine [11]. This innovation in nicotine chemistry is a critical factor in the addictiveness of pod mods like JUUL [11]. Because pod mods like JUUL are able to deliver highly addictive doses of nicotine without any adverse user experiences, 80% of youth and young adults who try JUUL continue using the product [52]. The safety of this form of nicotine, however, is unknown [8].

PROVIDER RECOMMENDATIONS

Health care providers can play a pivotal role in the prevention of ENDS use among youth. Youth generally see health care providers at least annually between the ages of 11 and 18 years [53]. In addition, youth often present for sick visits as well as visits for preparticipation examinations required when playing sports. All of these entry points into the health care system provide health care providers with the opportunity to screen for use and provide developmentally appropriate anticipatory guidance to youth and their families.

Screening/risk assessment methods

In its 2015 clinical practice policy, the American Association of Pediatrics (AAP) strongly recommended universal screening for the use of tobacco and exposure to tobacco smoke during all wellness visits and sick visits in which the chief complaint and diagnosis may be associated with tobacco smoke exposure [54]. The US Preventive Services Task Force has drafted a summary recommendation update urging primary care providers to use interventions to prevent tobacco use, including initiation of ENDS devices, to adolescents and school-aged children [55]. Despite these strong recommendations, the level of evidence for screening of tobacco use and exposure is deemed low, because of a lack of clinical trials supporting the efficacy of screening during clinic visits [56].

Many health care providers include screening for tobacco and ENDS use in the Previsit Questionnaire completed by the youth at the onset of an annual health supervision visit [53]. Health care providers should also consider discussing this risk behavior one on one during the visit. Many youth erroneously consider ENDS to be safe products without risk [53]. It may be of value to further clarify inherent risks. In addition, health care providers should consider asking about use of ENDS by family members and friends because youth and young adults are more likely to begin using ENDS if family and friends are ENDS users [53]. Youth and young adults who use ENDS are more likely to also use traditional cigarettes [53].

Many of the screening tools commonly used for substance use disorders in the pediatric population have not been adapted to specifically ask questions about ENDS use. Such tools include the S2BI (Screening to Brief Intervention) and the BSTAD (Brief Screener for Tobacco, Alcohol, and Other Drugs) [57]. The HEEADSSS (Home, Education/Employment, Eating, Activities, Drugs, Sexuality, Suicidal ideation and Safety) assessment tool for adolescents, an open-ended screening tool for risky behavior, can easily be modified to inquire about vaping behavior. This psychosocial screening interview requires about 15 minutes to administer and should be conducted in an area free of distraction [58]. Clinicians should modify their questions using terminology such as "vaping" and "e-cigs" because not all adolescents equate ENDS with smoking or tobacco use [54].

The most well-studied screening tool for substance use in adolescents from ages 12 to 21 is the Car, Relax, Alone, Forget, Friends, Trouble (CRAFFT) screening tool [59]. It has demonstrated validity among youth from diverse racial/ethnic and socioeconomic backgrounds [59]. Endorsed by the AAP's Bright Futures guidelines [53], the CRAFFT+N model begins with a question about tobacco and nicotine products, including e-cigarettes and vaping [59]. There are both self-administered and clinician-administered versions of this tool [59].

In addition to screening for use and susceptibility to use, health care providers should also consider screening youth who already use ENDS for nicotine dependence. The PROMIS-E (Patient-Reported Outcomes Measurement Information System Nicotine Dependence Item Bank for E-cigarettes) reliably assesses nicotine dependence in adolescent e-cigarette users [60]. This 4-item screen rapidly evaluates symptoms of dependence in self-identified ENDS users in the past month [60].

Many of these screening tools can be incorporated into the Previsit Questionnaire or the portion of the electronic heath record used during the visit. Many health care facilities, including primary care offices, emergency rooms, and urgent cares, have incorporated a general screening question about tobacco smoke use and/or exposure at the sick and well visit. These questions can be easily adapted to also include ENDS use and/or exposure.

Anticipatory guidance for parents and teens

The AAP clearly describes anticipatory guidance with regard to ENDS use for youth and their parents in the text, *Bright Futures: Guidelines for Health Supervision of Infants, Children, and Adolescents* [53]. The topic of ENDS use is introduced at the 11-year health supervision visit, although screening for tobacco and ENDS exposure in the home should begin much earlier [53]. Messaging specific to youth includes the following:

- Encouraging youth not to use ENDS
- Providing support for friends who choose not to use ENDS
- Choosing friends who support the youth's decision not to use ENDS, and
- Offering support to youth who are currently using ENDS who wish to discontinue use [53]

Messaging specific to parents of youth includes the following:

- Being knowledgeable about where and with whom their youth spends leisure time
- Discussing family rules about the use of ENDS with their youth, and
- Praising youth who are choosing not to use ENDS [53]

Health care professionals can make an impact just by providing clear, targeted messaging concerning ENDS use and exposure among youth to youth and their families.

SUMMARY

ENDS use among youth is on the increase and represents a risk for potentially toxic chemical exposures and the development of nicotine addiction. The understanding of the health effects of ENDS use on youth is still emerging, and there is an increasing need for research in this area. Given the inherent risks incurred with ENDS use during youth, it is imperative that health care professionals screen and provide targeted messages about ENDS use with youth and their families.

Disclosure

The authors report no conflicts of interest.

References

[1] Kholy KE, Genco RJ, Van Dyke TE. Oral infections and cardiovascular disease. Trends Endocrinol Metab 2015;26(6):315–21.
[2] US Department of Health and Human Services. E-cigarette use among youth and young adults. A report of the surgeon general. Atlanta (GA): US Department of Health and Human Services, Centers for Disease Control and Prevention, National Center for Chronic Disease Prevention and Health Promotion, Office on Smoking and Health; 2016.
[3] Glasser AM, Collins L, Pearson JL, et al. Overview of electronic nicotine delivery systems: a systematic review. Am J Prev Med 2017;52(2):e33–66.
[4] McMillen RC, Gottlieb MA, Shaefer RMW, et al. Trends in electronic cigarette use among US adults: use is increasing in both smokers and nonsmokers. Nicotine Tob Res 2014;17(10):1195–202.
[5] Jamal A, Gentzke A, Hu SS, et al. Tobacco use among middle and high school students—United States, 2011–2016. MMWR Morb Mortal Wkly Rep 2017;66(23):597.
[6] Gentzke AS, Creamer M, Cullen KA, et al. Vital signs: tobacco product use among middle and high school students—United States, 2011–2018. MMWR Morb Mortal Wkly Rep 2019;68(6):157.
[7] Arrazola RA, Singh T, Corey CG, et al. Tobacco use among middle and high school students—United States, 2011–2014. MMWR Morb Mortal Wkly Rep 2015;64(14):381.
[8] Truth initiative. E-cigarettes. 2018. Available at: https://truthinitiative.org/sites/default/files/media/files/2019/03/Truth_E-Cigarette_FactSheet_FINAL.pdf. Accessed September 12, 2019.
[9] Chen C, Zhuang Y-L, Zhu S-HJ. E-cigarette design preference and smoking cessation: a US population study. Am J Prev Med 2016;51(3):356–63.
[10] McEwen A, McRobbie H. Electronic cigarettes: a briefing for stop smoking services. United Kingdom: National Centre for Smoking Cessation and Training, Public Health England; 2016.

[11] Barrington-Trimis JL, Leventhal AM. Adolescents' use of "pod mod" e-cigarettes—urgent concerns. N Engl J Med 2018;379(12):1099–102.

[12] King BA, Patel R, Nguyen K, et al. Trends in awareness and use of electronic cigarettes among US adults, 2010-2013. Nicotine Tob Res 2015;17(2):219–27.

[13] Schoenborn CA, Clarke TC. QuickStats: percentage of adults who ever used an E-cigarette and percentage who currently use E-cigarettes, by age group—National Health Interview Survey, United States, 2016 (vol 66, pg 892, 2016). MMWR Morb Mortal Wkly Rep 2017;66(44):1238.

[14] Syamlal G. Electronic cigarette use among working adults—United States, 2014. MMWR Morb Mortal Wkly Rep 2016;65:557–61.

[15] Mirbolouk M, Charkhchi P, Orimoloye OA, et al. E-Cigarette use without a history of combustible cigarette smoking among U.S. adults: behavioral risk factor surveillance system, 2016. Ann Intern Med 2019;170(1):76–9.

[16] Zhu S-H, Sun JY, Bonnevie E, et al. Four hundred and sixty brands of e-cigarettes and counting: implications for product regulation. Tob Control 2014;23(suppl 3):iii3–9.

[17] Bhatnagar A, Whitsel LP, Ribisl KM, et al, American Heart Association Advocacy Coordinating Committee, Council on Cardiovascular and Stroke Nursing, Council on Clinical Cardiology, and Council on Quality of Care and Outcomes Research. Electronic cigarettes: a policy statement from the American Heart Association. Circulation 2014;130(16):1418–36.

[18] Loria K. Use of E-cigarettes among teens is 'exploding'. Consumer reports 2019. 2019. Available at: https://www.consumerreports.org/electronic-cigarettes/e-cigarette-use-among-teens-is-exploding/. Accessed September 12, 2019.

[19] Centers for Disease Control and Prevention. Quick facts on the risks of e-cigarettes for kids, teens, and young adults. Smoking & Tobacco Use 2019. 2019. Available at: https://www.cdc.gov/tobacco/basic_information/e-cigarettes/Quick-Facts-on-the-Risks-of-E-cigarettes-for-Kids-Teens-and-Young-Adults.html. Accessed August 24, 2019.

[20] White J, Li J, Newcombe R, et al. Tripling use of electronic cigarettes among New Zealand adolescents between 2012 and 2014. J Adolesc Health 2015;56(5):522–8.

[21] Kong G, Morean ME, Cavallo DA, et al. Reasons for electronic cigarette experimentation and discontinuation among adolescents and young adults. Nicotine Tob Res 2014;17(7):847–54.

[22] Peters RJ Jr, Meshack A, Lin M-T, et al. The social norms and beliefs of teenage male electronic cigarette use. J Ethn Subst Abuse 2013;12(4):300–7.

[23] Lippert AM. Do adolescent smokers use e-cigarettes to help them quit? The sociodemographic correlates and cessation motivations of US adolescent e-cigarette use. Am J Health Promot 2015;29(6):374–9.

[24] Breland A, Soule E, Lopez A, et al. Electronic cigarettes: what are they and what do they do? Ann N Y Acad Sci 2017;1394(1):5.

[25] Centers for Disease Control and Prevention (CDC). Tobacco product use among middle and high school students—United States, 2011 and 2012. MMWR Morb Mortal Wkly Rep 2013;62(45):893.

[26] Food and Drug Administration. Deeming tobacco products to be subject to the Federal Food, Drug, and Cosmetic Act, as amended by the Family Smoking Prevention and Tobacco Control Act; restrictions on the sale and distribution of tobacco products and required warning statements for tobacco products. Final rule. Fed Regist 2016;81(90):28973.

[27] LaVito A. FDA outlines e-cigarette rules, tightens restrictions on fruity flavors to try to curb teen vaping. CNBC Health and Science. 2019. Available at: https://www.cnbc.com/2019/03/13/fda-tightens-restrictions-on-flavored-e-cigarettes-to-curb-teen-vaping.html. Accessed October 15, 2019.

[28] Campaign for Tobacco Free Kids. States and localities that have raised the minimum legal sale age for tobacco products to 21. 2019. Available at: https://www.tobaccofreekids.org/

assets/content/what_we_do/state_local_issues/sales_21/states_localities_MLSA_21.pdf. Accessed August 24, 2019.

[29] U.S. Food & Drug Administration. FDA's youth tobacco prevention plan. Tobacco products. 2019. Available at: https://www.fda.gov/tobacco-products/youth-and-tobacco/fdas-youth-tobacco-prevention-plan. Accessed August 24, 2019.

[30] National Academies of Sciences, Engineering, and Medicine. Public health consequences of e-cigarettes. Washington, DC: The National Academies Press; 2018.

[31] Belkoniene M, Socquet J, Njemba-Freiburghaus D, et al. Near fatal intoxication by nicotine and propylene glycol injection: a case report of an e-liquid poisoning. BMC Pharmacol Toxicol 2019;20(1):28.

[32] Severe Pulmonary Disease Associated with using E-Cigarette Products [press release]. CDC Health Alert Network 2019.

[33] Centers for Disease Control and Prevention. How tobacco smoke causes disease: the biology and behavioral basis for smoking-attributable disease: a report from the surgeon general. Atlanta, GA: Centers for Disease Control and Prevention, National Center for Chronic Disease Prevention and Health Promotion, Office on Smoking and Health; 2010.

[34] Yuan M, Cross SJ, Loughlin SE. Nicotine and the adolescent brain. J Physiol 2015;593(16): 3397–412.

[35] Allen JG, Flanigan SS, LeBlanc M, et al. Flavoring chemicals in e-cigarettes: diacetyl, 2,3-pentanedione, and acetoin in a sample of 51 products, including fruit-, candy-, and cocktail-flavored e-cigarettes. Environ Health Perspect 2016;124(6):733.

[36] Bein K, Leikauf GD. Acrolein–a pulmonary hazard. Mol Nutr Food Res 2011;55(9): 1342–60.

[37] Herrington JS, Myers C. Electronic cigarette solutions and resultant aerosol profiles. J Chromatogr A 2015;1418:192–9.

[38] Fagan P, Pokhrel P, Herzog TA, et al. Sugar and aldehyde content in flavored electronic cigarette liquids. Nicotine Tob Res 2018;20(8):985–92.

[39] Clapp PW, Pawlak EA, Lackey JT, et al. Flavored e-cigarette liquids and cinnamaldehyde impair respiratory innate immune cell function. Am J Physiol Lung Cell Mol Physiol 2017;313(2):L278–92.

[40] Salathe M, Garcia-Arcos I, Geraghty P, et al. Nicotine in electronic-cigarettes causes inflammation, airway hyperreactivity and lung tissue destruction. American Journal of Respiratory and Critical Care Medicine 2015;191:A4030.

[41] Brass DM, Gwinn WM, Valente AM, et al. The diacetyl-exposed human airway epithelial secretome: new insights into flavoring-induced airways disease. Am J Respir Cell Mol Biol 2017;56(6):784–95.

[42] Orr MS. Electronic cigarettes in the USA: a summary of available toxicology data and suggestions for the future. Tob Control 2014;23(suppl 2):ii18–22.

[43] Barrington-Trimis JL, Samet JM, McConnell R. Flavorings in electronic cigarettes: an unrecognized respiratory health hazard? JAMA 2014;312(23):2493–4.

[44] Cheng T. Chemical evaluation of electronic cigarettes. Tob Control 2014;23(suppl 2): ii11–7.

[45] Kosmider L, Sobczak A, Fik M, et al. Carbonyl compounds in electronic cigarette vapors: effects of nicotine solvent and battery output voltage. Nicotine Tob Res 2014;16(10): 1319–26.

[46] Jensen RP, Luo W, Pankow JF, et al. Hidden formaldehyde in e-cigarette aerosols. N Engl J Med 2015;2015(372):392–4.

[47] Erythropel HC, Jabba SV, DeWinter TM, et al. Formation of flavorant-propylene glycol adducts with novel toxicological properties in chemically unstable E-cigarette liquids. Nicotine Tob Res 2019;21(9):1248–58.

[48] Williams M, Villarreal A, Bozhilov K, et al. Metal and silicate particles including nanoparticles are present in electronic cigarette cartomizer fluid and aerosol. PLoS One 2013;8(3): e57987.

[49] Saffari A, Daher N, Ruprecht A, et al. Particulate metals and organic compounds from electronic and tobacco-containing cigarettes: comparison of emission rates and secondhand exposure. Environ Sci Process Impacts 2014;16(10):2259–67.

[50] Lerner CA, Sundar IK, Yao H, et al. Vapors produced by electronic cigarettes and e-juices with flavorings induce toxicity, oxidative stress, and inflammatory response in lung epithelial cells and in mouse lung. PLoS One 2015;10(2):e0116732.

[51] Schweitzer KS, Chen SX, Law S, et al. Endothelial disruptive proinflammatory effects of nicotine and e-cigarette vapor exposures. Am J Physiol Lung Cell Mol Physiol 2015;309(2): L175–87.

[52] Willett JG, Bennett M, Hair EC, et al. Recognition, use and perceptions of JUUL among youth and young adults. Tob Control 2019;28(1):115–6.

[53] Hagan J, Shaw J, Duncan P, editors. Bright futures: guidelines for health supervision of Infants, children, and adolescents. 4th edition. Elk Grove Village (IL): American Academy of Pediatrics; 2017.

[54] Farber HJ, Walley SC, Groner JA, et al. Clinical practice policy to protect children from tobacco, nicotine, and tobacco smoke. Pediatrics 2015;136(5):1008–17.

[55] US Preventive Services Task Force. Draft recommendation statement: prevention and cessation of tobacco use in children and adolescents: primary care interventions. 2019. Available at: https://www.uspreventiveservicestaskforce.org/Page/Document/draft-recommendation-statement/tobacco-and-nicotine-use-prevention-in-children-and-adolescents-primary-care-interventions. Accessed September 13, 2019.

[56] Tanksi S, Garfunkel LC, Duncan PM, et al, editors. Preforming preventative services: a bright futures handbook. Elk Grove Village (IL): American Academy of Pediatrics; 2010.

[57] National Institute on Drug Abuse. Screening tools and prevention. Available at: https://www.drugabuse.gov/nidamed-medical-health-professionals/screening-tools-prevention. Accessed September 13, 2019.

[58] Doukrou M, Segal TY. Fifteen-minute consultation: communicating with young people–how to use HEEADSSS, a psychosocial interview for adolescents. Arch Dis Child Educ Pract Ed 2018;103(1):15–9.

[59] Knight JR, Harris SK, Sherritt L, et al. About the CRAFFT. 2018. Available at: https://crafft.org/about-us/.

[60] Morean ME, Krishnan-Sarin S, S O'Malley S. Assessing nicotine dependence in adolescent E-cigarette users: the 4-item patient-reported outcomes measurement information system (PROMIS) nicotine dependence item bank for electronic cigarettes. Drug Alcohol Depend 2018;188:60–3.

Advances in Family Practice Nursing 2 (2020) 159–168

ADVANCES IN FAMILY PRACTICE NURSING

ELSEVIER
MOSBY

Autism Spectrum Disorder in the Primary Care Setting

Importance of Early Diagnosis and Intervention

Susan Brasher, PhD, MSN, CPNP-PC[a],*,
Jennifer L. Stapel-Wax, PsyD[b]

[a]Emory University, Nell Hodgson Woodruff School of Nursing, 1520 Clifton Road Northeast, Atlanta, GA 30322, USA; [b]Department of Pediatrics, Emory University, Infant Toddler Community Outreach, Marcus Autism Center, Children's Healthcare of Atlanta, 1920 Briarcliff Road Northeast, Atlanta, GA 30329, USA

Keywords

• Autism spectrum disorder • Infants • Toddlers • Screening • Detection • Diagnosis
• Early • Intervention

Key points

• Maximizing early brain development sets the foundation for optimal outcomes across the life span.

• Early and consistent screening for diversions from typical development facilitates early action on delays in infants and toddlers.

• Autism spectrum disorder (ASD) is a disorder with profound impact on early brain development.

• There are recognizable early red flags of social communication deficits as well as consistent screening measures that can reliably discern and facilitate identification of children with ASD.

• It is paramount that very young children receive critical early intervention to maximize their development and enhance developmental outcomes.

INTRODUCTION

Autism spectrum disorder (ASD) is a complex neurodevelopmental disorder characterized by impairments in socialization and communication, as well as the presence of restricted and repetitive behaviors, interests, or activities [1]. Early diagnosis and subsequent treatment with evidence-based interventions

*Corresponding author. E-mail address: Susan.n.brasher@emory.edu
Twitter: @susanb59 (S.B.); @drjlsw (J.L.S.-W.)

https://doi.org/10.1016/j.yfpn.2020.01.006
2589-420X/20/© 2020 Elsevier Inc. All rights reserved.

have been linked to improved long-term outcomes and prognosis of children with ASD [2–6]. Although a reliable ASD diagnosis can be achieved by age 2 years, the current average age of ASD diagnosis in the United States is between 4 and 5 years and is later in select racial, ethnic, and gender minority populations [7–10].

ASD is a lifelong developmental disability associated with significant social, communication, and behavioral challenges [11]. At present, it is estimated that 1 in 59 children are diagnosed with ASD at 8 years of age [7,12]. Given the life-long implications and impact early diagnosis and intervention have on the developmental trajectory of individuals with ASD, early detection has become a public health concern [13]. Despite these facts, ASD screening rates in the United States remain low and a sizable gap persists between when a child can be diagnosed with ASD compared with the age of actual diagnosis [14]. Of particular concern are reports indicating that 85% of children with ASD had parental concerns noted in their medical record, whereas only 42% of those children had received a developmental evaluation [15]. Therefore, this article outlines the importance of early ASD diagnosis and intervention, as well as providing resources for family nurse practitioners (FNPs) to use in their practices.

EARLY BRAIN DEVELOPMENT

The period of birth to 3 years of age is a time of tremendous early brain development and change [16,17]. During this time, brain architecture and processing advance at a rapid rate. Given these implications, diversions from typical development, if recognized early, can result in early intervention and produce meaningful changes to a child's developmental trajectory [2,3,5]. Specifically, earlier diagnosis and intervention have been linked to enhanced IQ (intelligence quotient), expressive and receptive language gains, and improved adaptive behavior [2,6]. Studies have found that children who received an earlier ASD diagnosis and subsequent earlier intervention had a measurable decrease in ASD symptom severity [2,3,5,6].

AUTISM SYMPTOMS

Symptoms of ASD emerge in early childhood, with parental concerns reported as early as 6 to 12 months old [8,18,19]. Potential red flags for ASD include children not responding to their names by 12 months old, lack of pointing at objects by 14 months old, absence of pretend play by 18 months old, avoiding eye contact, and preferring to play alone (Boxes 1 and 2) [11]. Several tools exist to help parents and primary care providers understand the signs and symptoms of ASD, including the Autism Navigator, Learn the Signs Act Early, and Autism Initiatives (Tables 1 and 2) [20–22].

BROAD DEVELOPMENTAL SCREENING

Current recommendations support routine developmental surveillance by all primary care providers at well-child visits beginning at 9 months old [11,23]. Broad developmental screening tools (Box 3) identify delays in development

Box 1: Potential red flags for autism spectrum disorder for children 12 to 18 months old

Lack of appropriate gaze

Lack of warm, joyful expressions with gaze

Lack of sharing enjoyment or interest

Lack of response to name

Lack of coordination of gaze, facial expression, gesture, and sound

Lack of showing gestures

Unusual prosody (ie, inability to vary pitch, loudness, tempo, and rhythm in speech)

Repetitive movements or posturing of body, arms, hands, or fingers

Repetitive movements with objects

Data from Wetherby AM, Woods J, Allen L, Cleary J, Dickinson H, Lord C. Early Indicators of autism spectrum disorders in the second year of life. *J Autism Dev Disord.* 2004;34(5):473-493. https://doi.org/10.1007/s10803-004-2544-y.

Box 2: Potential red flags for autism spectrum disorder for children 18 to 24 months old

Trouble understanding other people's feelings

Difficulty talking about their feelings

Delayed speech and language skills, including language regression or loss of words

Repeats words or phrases (echolalia)

Gives unrelated answers to questions

Upset by minor changes and does not handle change well

Flaps hands, rocks body back and forth, or spins circles

Interest in watching objects spin

Unusual reactions to sound, smell, taste, or feel

Avoids or resists physical contact

Flat or inappropriate facial expressions

Talks in a flat, monotone, or sing-song voice

Lines up toys or other objects

Failure of back-and-forth conversation

Failure to initiate or respond to social interactions

Data from CDC. Learn the signs. Act early. https://www.cdc.gov/ncbddd/actearly/index.html. Published May 3, 2019. Accessed September 18, 2019.

Table 1
Educational tools about early brain development and autism spectrum disorder for primary care providers

Tool/web site	Location
Autism Navigator for Primary Care	https://autismnavigator.com/autism-navigator-for-primary-care/: 8-h course on early signs of ASD, including early screening, detection, and referral Cost: $625.00
First Words Project	https://firstwordsproject.com
CDC Autism Information	https://www.cdc.gov/ncbddd/autism/index.html
CDC Learn the Signs Act Early	https://www.cdc.gov/ncbddd/actearly/index.html
Zero to Three	https://www.zerotothree.org
Harvard Center for the Developing Child	https://developingchild.harvard.edu
American Academy of Pediatrics STAR	https://www.aap.org/en-us/advocacy-and-policy/aap-health-initiatives/Screening/: free resources on screening recommendations, tools, interactive training, and practice success stories

Abbreviations: CDC, US Centers for Disease Control and Prevention; STAR, Screening Technical Assistance & Resource Center.
Data from Refs [21,30–35].

Table 2
Educational tools about early brain development and autism spectrum disorder for families

Tool/web site	Location
Autism Navigator	http://autismnavigator.com
First Words Project	http://firstwordsproject.com
CDC Learn the Signs Act Early	https://www.cdc.gov/ncbddd/actearly/index.html
Talk With Me Baby	http://www.talkwithmebaby.org
Baby Navigator	https://babynavigator.com
First Signs	http://www.firstsigns.org
Zero to Three	https://www.zerotothree.org

Data from Refs [20,21,31,33,36–38].

Box 3: Broad developmental screening tools

Ages and Stages Questionnaire (ASQ)

Communication and Symbolic Behavior Scales Developmental Profile (CSBS DP) and Infant Toddler Checklist (ITC)

Parents' Evaluation of Developmental Status (PEDS)

Data from Refs [39–41].

but are not considered to be specific to autism. They are highly valid and reliable in detecting deficits in communication, gross-motor, fine-motor, problem-solving, and social-emotional development [24].

AUTISM-SPECIFIC SCREENING

Beginning at the 18-month well-child visit, primary care providers are recommended to screen all children specifically for ASD using validated and reliable ASD screening tools [11,23]. These screening tools can be categorized as level 1 screening tools and level 2 screening tools. Level 1 screening tools (Table 3) are intended to screen all children for ASD and are considered to be universal ASD screeners. In contrast, level 2 screening tools (see Table 3) are intended to be used specifically for children who are at increased risk for ASD

Table 3
Autism spectrum disorder–specific screening tools

Screening tool	Type of screener	Information
M-CHAT-R/F	Level 1	Parent questionnaire 20 items Time: 5–10 min Free If delays or deviations are noted, a follow-up interview about those items by the clinician is needed to verify the noted behavior
POSI	Level 1	The POSI is an autism-specific screener that is a subscale within the SWYC Parent questionnaire 10–17 items, 5-point Likert rating scale from never to many times a day Time: 5–10 min Free
STAT	Level 2	Interactive provider observational method 12 activities 20 min Cost: $500 per kit
SORF	Level 2	Interactive provider observational method
BISCUIT	Level 2	Composed of 3 separate measures, including interactive provider observational method
DBC-ES	Level 2	Parent report 17 items 5–10 min 0, 1, 2 rating (0, not true as far as is known; 1, somewhat or sometimes true; 2, very true or often true) Cost: $147

Abbreviations: BISCUIT, baby and infant screen for children with autism traits; DBC-ES, the developmental behavior checklist–early screen; M-CHAT-R/F, modified checklist for autism in toddlers; POSI, parent's observations of social interactions; SORF, systematic observation of red flags of ASD; STAT, screening tool for autism in toddlers and young children; SWYC, survey of well-being of young children.
Data from Refs [29,42–46].

because of family history and heightened parent/provider concerns [14]. Note that although a wide range of validated and reliable level 1 and level 2 ASD screening tools exist, the Modified Checklist for Autism in Toddlers (M-CHAT) and subsequent revised follow-up screening (M-CHAT R/F) is considered to be the most commonly studied and widely used autism screening tool [25].

THE ROLE OF THE FAMILY NURSE PRACTITIONER IN EARLY AUTISM DIAGNOSIS AND INTERVENTION

As primary care providers, FNPs play a critical role in evaluating childhood development and are thus well positioned to detect signs of ASD at a very early age. As a member of the nation's most trusted profession, parents look to FNPs with questions and concerns for their children's development. FNPs have a great opportunity to shape children's developmental trajectory not only through developmental surveillance and screening but also by engaging parents in discussions about concerns for their children's development. One way in which FNPs can do this is by consistently asking parents at every visit whether they have any concerns about their children's behavior or development [15]. By having these conversations regularly, FNPs can create an opening for parents to share their developmental concerns and alert the FNP to critical next steps. Regardless of the FNPs' educational training backgrounds, all FNPs are able to access autism-specific resources and tools to enhance their awareness of ASD (see Table 1). FNPs should refer to the US Centers for Disease Control and Prevention (CDC) Pediatric Developmental Screening Flowchart (Fig. 1) to guide them on the ASD-specific screening process and steps to take when a child screens negative or positive [11].

OBSTACLES TO SCREENING

Despite growing awareness and recognition of the importance of early ASD diagnosis and treatment, obstacles have been noted to exist in the clinical setting that could affect clinicians' ability or willingness to complete autism screening. Studies have reported that the leading reasons for not routinely performing ASD screening were insufficient time to screen, unfamiliarity with screening tools, lack of reimbursement, and cost of screening tools [14,26].

OVERCOMING OBSTACLES TO SCREENING

Several strategies have been identified to overcome obstacles to screening. Included in these strategies are training of health care providers at all levels, better education of providers, involvement of staff and parents in the screening process, access to evidence-based screening tools, and alternative delivery format of screening tools (eg, electronic delivery before visit, use of technology to complete screening tools in waiting room) [14].

The use of Current Procedural Terminology (CPT) codes are an effective way to overcome obstacles to screening caused by cost and insufficient time. The CPT code 96110 is commonly used when deploying limited

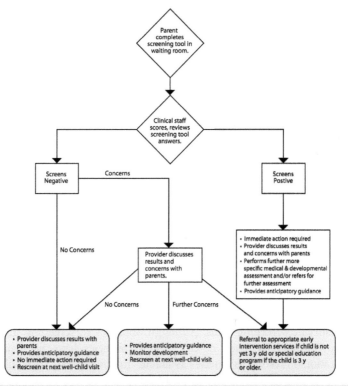

Fig. 1. Pediatric developmental screening flowchart. (*From* CDC. Signs & symptoms. Autism spectrum disorder (ASD). Centers for Disease Control and Prevention. https://www.cdc.gov/ncbddd/autism/hcp-screening.html. Published February 26, 2015. Accessed September 18, 2019.)

developmental testing, including screening tools listed in Box 3 and Table 3. This code is frequently used during preventive medical services but may also be used when screening is performed during acute services (eg, illness, follow-up visits) [27]. Alternatively, the CPT code 961111 is commonly used when deploying longer, more comprehensive developmental testing that requires direct observation with tools such as those listed in Table 3.

SUMMARY

Often the earliest signs of developmental deviation are subtle and difficult to fully differentiate as a diagnosable disorder. Therefore, the knowledge of primary care providers is integral to the success of recognizing developmental delays and providing a pathway to early diagnosis and intervention in young children. Having a solid foundation of knowledge on early brain development and the social and communication milestones in the first 2 years of life is profoundly important to the goal of effective screening and detection. This foundation also provides clinicians the necessary confidence in relaying their clinical opinions to the parents and can greatly expedite referral for early diagnosis and intervention.

Best-practice recommendations highlight 2 important strategies FNPs can use to reduce the age of ASD diagnosis: broad developmental screenings and ASD-specific screenings. The American Academy of Pediatrics and Bright Futures encourages clinicians to engage in routine developmental surveillance of all patients beginning at 9 months old followed by a targeted ASD-specific screening at 18 months old [23]. Although the practice of routine developmental surveillance enhances the outcomes for all children, the use of ASD-specific screening tools can assist in early detection of ASD, earlier referral for diagnosis, and access to evidence-based interventions [14,28].

Research has established that birth to 3 years of age is a critical point in early childhood development and one at which it is imperative to detect diversions from typical development in order to implement early intervention [2,3,5]. Early ASD diagnosis and intervention have been shown to enhance children's developmental trajectory, thus improving long-term outcomes [4,13].

FNPs are among the most trusted professionals and on the frontline of recognizing early childhood development deviations. It is important for FNPs to be familiar with potential red flags for ASD, broad developmental screening tools, and ASD-specific screening tools. Although obstacles to screening in the primary care setting have been noted, several strategies have been proposed and educational resources made available to overcome such obstacles. Through the use of such strategies and resources, FNPs have the opportunity to close the gap of age in diagnosis of ASD.

Disclosure

The authors have nothing to disclose.

References

[1] American Psychological Association. Diagnostic and statistical manual of mental disorders. 5th edition. Washington, DC: APA; 2013.

[2] Dawson G, Rogers S, Munson J, et al. Randomized, controlled trial of an intervention for toddlers with autism: the Early Start Denver model. Pediatrics 2010;125(1):e17–23.

[3] Green J, Pickles A, Pasco G, et al. Randomised trial of a parent-mediated intervention for infants at high risk for autism: longitudinal outcomes to age 3 years. J Child Psychol Psychiatry 2017;58(12):1330–40.

[4] Koegel LK, Koegel RL, Ashbaugh K, et al. The importance of early identification and intervention for children with or at risk for autism spectrum disorders. Int J Speech Lang Pathol 2014;16(1):50–6.

[5] Pickles A, Le Couteur A, Leadbitter K, et al. Parent-mediated social communication therapy for young children with autism (PACT): long-term follow-up of a randomised controlled trial. Lancet 2016;388(10059):2501–9.

[6] Rogers SJ, Vismara L, Wagner AL, et al. Autism treatment in the first year of life: a pilot study of Infant Start, a parent-implemented intervention for symptomatic infants. J Autism Dev Disord 2014;44(12):2981–95.

[7] Baio J, Wiggins L, Christensen DL, et al. Prevalence of autism spectrum disorder among children aged 8 years — autism and developmental disabilities monitoring network, 11 Sites, United States, 2014. MMWR Surveill Summ 2018;67(6):1–23.

[8] Lord C, Risi S, DiLavore PS, et al. Autism from 2 to 9 years of age. Arch Gen Psychiatry 2006;63(6):694.

[9] Mandell DS, Wiggins LD, Carpenter LA, et al. Racial/ethnic disparities in the identification of children with autism spectrum disorders. Am J Public Health 2009;99(3):493–8.

[10] Zwaigenbaum L, Bauman ML, Stone WL, et al. Early identification of autism spectrum disorder: recommendations for practice and research. Pediatrics 2015;136(Supplement): S10–40.

[11] CDC. Signs & symptoms. Autism spectrum disorder (ASD). Centers for Disease Control and Prevention. 2015. Available at: https://www.cdc.gov/ncbddd/autism/hcp-screening.html. Accessed September 18, 2019.

[12] CDC. Data and statistics on autism spectrum disorder. Centers for Disease Control and Prevention. 2019. Available at: https://www.cdc.gov/ncbddd/autism/data.html. Accessed September 16, 2019.

[13] Sturner R, Howard B, Bergmann P, et al. Comparison of autism screening in younger and older toddlers. J Autism Dev Disord 2017;47(10):3180–8.

[14] Zwaigenbaum L, Bauman ML, Fein D, et al. Early screening of autism spectrum disorder: recommendations for practice and research. Pediatrics 2015;136(Supplement):S41–59.

[15] Jenco M. CDC: autism rates increase slightly to 1 in 59 children. AAP News; 2019. Available at: https://www.aappublications.org/news/2018/04/26/autism042618. Accessed September 18, 2019.

[16] The National Early Childhood Technical Assistance Center. The importance of early intervention. 2011. Available at: https://ectacenter.org/pubs/pubdetails.asp?pubsid=104. Accessed September 28, 2019.

[17] Harvard University. Brain architecture. 2017. Available at: https://developingchild.harvard.edu/science/key-concepts/brain-architecture/. Accessed September 28, 2019.

[18] Elder J, Kreider C, Brasher S, et al. Clinical impact of early diagnosis of autism on the prognosis and parent-child relationships. Psychol Res Behav Manag 2017;10:283–92.

[19] Sacrey L-AR, Zwaigenbaum L, Bryson S, et al. Can parents' concerns predict autism spectrum disorder? a prospective study of high-risk siblings from 6 to 36 months of age. J Am Acad Child Adolesc Psychiatry 2015;54(6):470–8.

[20] Autism Navigator. Autism navigator. 2019. Available at: http://autismnavigator.com/. Accessed September 28, 2019.

[21] CDC. Learn the signs. Act early. 2019. Available at: https://www.cdc.gov/ncbddd/actearly/index.html. Accessed September 18, 2019.

[22] AAP. Autism Initiatives. 2019. Available at: http://www.aap.org/en-us/advocacy-and-policy/aap-health-initiatives/Pages/autism-initiatives.aspx. Accessed September 18, 2019.

[23] AAP/Bright Futures. Recommendations for preventive pediatric healthcare. 2019. Available at: https://www.aap.org/en-us/Documents/periodicity_schedule.pdf. Accessed September 18, 2019.

[24] AAP. Screening tools. 2017. Available at: https://screeningtime.org/star-center/#/screening-tools. Accessed September 28, 2019.

[25] United States Preventive Services Task (USPSTF). Autism spectrum disorder in young children: screening. 2019. Available at: https://www.uspreventiveservicestaskforce.org/Page/Document/UpdateSummaryFinal/autism-spectrum-disorder-in-young-children-screening. Accessed September 28, 2019.

[26] Elder JH, Brasher S, Alexander B. Identifying the barriers to early diagnosis and treatment in underserved individuals with autism spectrum disorders (ASD) and their families: a qualitative study. Issues Ment Health Nurs 2016;37(6):412–20.

[27] AAP. Developmental screening/testing: coding fact sheet for primary care pediatricians. 2005. Available at: https://www.cdc.gov/ncbddd/autism/documents/AAP-Coding-Fact-Sheet-for-Primary-Care.pdf. Accessed September 24, 2019.

[28] Dosreis S, Weiner CL, Johnson L, et al. Autism spectrum disorder screening and management practices among general pediatric providers. J Dev Behav Pediatr 2006;27(Supplement 2):S88–94.

[29] Wetherby AM, Woods J, Allen L, et al. Early indicators of autism spectrum disorders in the second year of life. J Autism Dev Disord 2004;34(5):473–93.

[30] Autism navigator. Autism navigator for primary care. Available at: https://autismnavigator.com/autism-navigator-for-primary-care/.

[31] First Words Project. First words project. 2019. Available at: https://firstwordsproject.com. Accessed September 18, 2019.

[32] CDC. Autism spectrum disorder (ASD). 2019. Available at: https://www.cdc.gov/ncbddd/autism/index.html. Accessed September 28, 2019.

[33] Zero to three. Zero to three: early connections last a lifetime. 2019. Available at: https://www.zerotothree.org. Accessed September 28, 2019.

[34] Harvard University Center on the Developing Child. Reaching for breakthroughs with science-based innovations. 2019. Available at: https://developingchild.harvard.edu. Accessed September 28, 2019.

[35] AAP. Screening Technical Assistance and Resource (STAR) center. 2019. Available at: https://www.aap.org/en-us/advocacy-and-policy/aap-health-initiatives/Screening/Pages/default.aspx. Accessed September 18, 2019.

[36] Talk With Me Baby. Talk with me baby. 2019. Available at: http://www.talkwithmebaby.org. Accessed September 25, 2019.

[37] Baby Navigator. Baby navigator. 2019. Available at: https://babynavigator.com. Accessed September 28, 2019.

[38] First signs. First signs. 2016. Available at: http://www.firstsigns.org. Accessed September 28, 2019.

[39] Squires J, Bricker D. Ages & stages questionnaires (ASQ). 3rd edition. Brookes Publishing; 2009. Available at: http://www.agesandstages.com.

[40] Wetherby AM, Brosnan-Maddox S, Peace V, et al. Validation of the Infant—Toddler Checklist as a broadband screener for autism spectrum disorders from 9 to 24 months of age. Autism 2008;12(5):487–511.

[41] Glascoe FP. Parents' evaluation of developmental status. Nashville (TN): Ellsworth & Vandermeer Press, Ltd.; 1997.

[42] Robins DL, Barton M, Fein D. Modified checklist for autism in toddlers, revised with follow-up 2018; https://doi.org/10.1037/t67574-000.

[43] Floating Hospital for Children at Tufts Medical Center. Parent's Observations of Social Interactions (POSI). 2017. Available at: https://www.floatinghospital.org/The-Survey-of-Well-being-of-Young-Children/Parts-of-the-SWYC/POSI. Accessed September 18, 2019.

[44] Stone WL, McMahon CR, Henderson LM. Use of the Screening Tool for Autism in Two-year-olds (STAT) for children under 24 months: an exploratory study. Autism 2008;12(5):557–73.

[45] Matson JL, Wilkins J, Fodstad JC. The validity of the baby and infant screen for children with autism traits: part 1 (BISCUIT: Part 1). J Autism Dev Disord 2011;41(9):1139–46.

[46] Gray KM, Tonge BJ, Sweeney DJ, et al. Screening for autism in young children with developmental delay: an evaluation of the Developmental Behaviour Checklist: early Screen. J Autism Dev Disord 2008;38(6):1003–10.

Advances in Family Practice Nursing 2 (2020) 169–186

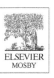

ADVANCES IN FAMILY PRACTICE NURSING

Human Trafficking in the Clinical Setting

Critical Competencies for Family Nurse Practitioners

Jessica L. Peck, DNP, APRN, CPNP-PC, CNE, CNL, FAANP

Louise Herrington School of Nursing, Baylor University, 333 North Washington Avenue, Dallas, TX 75246, USA

Keywords
- Human trafficking • Labor trafficking • Sex trafficking • Vulnerable
- Nurse practitioner • Trauma-informed care • Cultural responsiveness

Key points

- Family nurse practitioners may encounter trafficking victims and can serve as an important link in identification, connection to recovery services, and advocacy and prevention efforts.
- Misperceptions exist among health care providers about human trafficking, which facilitate its covert nature, making it critical to develop competencies aiding in trauma-informed victim identification and response.
- Health impacts of trafficking are multifaceted, including poorly managed chronic medical conditions, significant mental health issues, substance abuse/misuse, sexual health problems, and diminished life.
- Multidisciplinary holistic response in development of care models and organizational protocols is important for clinical care, case management, referral, and care coordination of trafficking victims.
- Health care can be an effective first responder force to raise awareness through evidence-based education, advocating for policy change, and implementing prevention measures for identified risk.

INTRODUCTION

Human trafficking (HT) is a ubiquitous global human rights violation rising in societal consciousness to the level of emerging humanitarian and public health

E-mail address: Jessica_Peck@Baylor.edu
Twitter: @DrPeckPNP (J.L.P.)

https://doi.org/10.1016/j.yfpn.2020.01.011
2589-420X/20/

crisis [1]. More than 40 million people are estimated to be currently victimized by HT worldwide [2]. Precise estimates of incidence and prevalence of HT in the United States are in the infancy stages of development, to a certain extent because of challenges intrinsic in effectuating scientific research amid a criminal enterprise with the hidden character of victimization and a complex maze of legal, cultural, and organizational barriers. Other challenges include lack of uniform, standardized terms and a centralized database for data collection and analysis [3]. Current estimates implicate the United States as a leading origin country for federally identified trafficking victims of all ages [4]. In 2018, the National Human Trafficking Hotline reported calls either directly from or regarding HT victims or survivors, including 10,731 adult reports; 4945 child reports (up from 2762 the year prior); and 7402 reports concerning victims of unknown age [5]. Although there is no official estimate of the number of HT victims in the United States, Polaris estimates the total number of victims spans the hundreds of thousands when considerations for adult and minor victims are aggregated collectively in both sex trafficking (ST) and labor trafficking (LT) estimates [6], with the largest numbers coming from California, Texas, Florida, Ohio, and New York [7]. Children are particularly vulnerable to entry into trafficking. Using the best data available, the International Labour Organization estimates children account for approximately 1 in 4 of the 21 million global victims of forced labor [8]. In addition, the United Nations Office of Drugs and Crime found 33% of 40,000 identified victims of trafficking were children [4]. Women and girls make up approximately 99% of victims in the commercial sex industry and 58% of victims in other sectors, including forced labor [8].

HT (sometimes referred to as modern-day slavery) is the most rapidly growing criminal industry in the world and second in revenue only to the drug trade [7]. Exploitation of human victims enables traffickers to make continuous profits with less risk compared with the criminal sale of consumable commodities, such as illicit drugs or guns, contributing to an estimated $150 billion annual revenue worldwide [9]. Up to 88% of victims report encountering at least 1 health care provider (HCP) while actively experiencing HT victimization without being identified [10]. Misconceptions persist among HCPs about the nature of HT and characteristics of victims [11]. Stereotyping victims and perpetrators can contribute to lack of timely identification and appropriate response [12].

Family nurse practitioners (FNPs) and other HCPs may encounter victims of HT in their clinical practices and can serve as an important link in identification of victimization and connection to recovery services as well as aiding in advocacy and prevention efforts [13]. The objectives of this article are to (1) understand the nature and scope of HT in the United States, (2) equip FNPs to identify potential signs of HT in victims who present for care in a medical setting, (3) integrate principles of trauma-informed care when caring for potentially trafficked persons, (4) implement multidisciplinary care models to aid in victim response and recovery, and (5) explore the clinician role in prevention, treatment, advocacy, and aftercare.

HISTORY

The Trafficking Victims Protection Act was established in 2000 to define HT legally at the federal level (Table 1) and is crucial in providing protection for victims as well as aiding in the prosecution of traffickers [14]. The action-means-purpose model (Fig. 1) illustrates this legal construct with the important distinction that minor victims under 16 years of age are considered victims of HT regardless of the presence of force, fraud, or coercion. Minors ages 17 or 18 do not have to prove force, fraud, or coercion if their trafficker is a person with authority over them (eg, parent, relative, teacher, employer, coach, or minister) [15,16]. There are 2 prevalent types of HT in the United States: (1) LT and (2) ST [16], for child victims, also referred to as commercial sexual exploitation of a child (CSEC) or domestic minor ST (DMST) [17]. Although ST often receives more awareness efforts and media attention, yielding visceral emotional response from the public at large, LT is an equally significant issue in the United States and should not be neglected in antitrafficking efforts and education initiatives for HCPs [18]. Many contributing factors help fuel HT as a criminal industry, including (1) high reward in securing lucrative economic profits and relatively low risk for criminal prosecution; (2) high demand from consumers for inexpensive goods requiring cheap labor (LT) and increased demand for commercial sex, incentivizing traffickers to recruit and exploit vulnerable individuals including children (ST, DMST, and CSEC); and (3) system inequalities and disparities in social determinants of health, such as conflict, poverty, decreased access to education, lack of employment opportunity, forced child marriage, and violence, all of which increase vulnerability for HT demand [19].

Many misperceptions exist among HCPs about HT, which facilitate enabling its covert nature and failure to identify potential victims (Box 1). Despite persistent public misperception of ST occurring only through forced prostitution, ST also occurs in pornography production, escort services, exotic dancing, and massage parlors, among others. Other misconceptions diminish awareness of and concern for LT in the United States [20]. Traffickers (commonly referred to as pimps, with the term often conveying undeserved societal glorification) are

Table 1	
Trafficking Victims Protection Act definitions	
Sex trafficking	Labor trafficking
The recruitment, harboring, transportation, provision, or obtaining of a person for the purpose of a commercial sex act, in which a commercial sex act is induced by force, fraud, or coercion, or in which the person forced to perform such an act is under the age of 18 y	The recruitment, harboring, transportation, provision, or obtaining of a person for labor or services, through the use of force, fraud, or coercion for the purpose of subjection to involuntary servitude, peonage, debt bondage or slavery

Data from The United States Department of Justice. Human Trafficking Defined. Available at: https://www.justice.gov/humantrafficking.

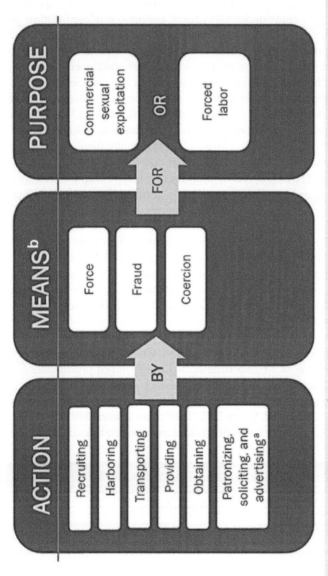

Fig. 1. The action-means-purpose model. [a] ST only. [b] Minors induced into commercial sex are HT victims, regardless if force, fraud, or coercion is present. (*Data from* Office on Trafficking in Persons. What is human trafficking? 2019. Available at: https://www.acf.hhs.gov/otip/about/what-is-human-trafficking. Accessed September 19, 2019.)

Box 1: Common myths about human trafficking

HT occurs mainly overseas.

Only foreign nationals are impacted.

HT is the same thing as human smuggling.

ST does not occur in legal businesses.

Prostitutes engage in sex work by choice.

Victims of HT will accept help when offered.

Only women and girls are victimized.

Child trafficking would never happen in my community.

All pimps look the same.

ST is the only kind of trafficking in the United States.

Data from the American Hospital Association. Dispelling myths about human trafficking for health care providers. 2018. Available at: https://www.aha.org/news/insights-and-analysis/2018-01-05-dispelling-myths-about-human-trafficking-health-care. Retrieved September 19, 2019.

serial predators who intentionally target vulnerable individuals. They often are willing to invest significant amounts of time into grooming efforts, knowing the potential lucrative financial profits awaiting [21]. It is important for HCPs to discard societal stereotypes or archetype images of traffickers, because they can and do present as men, women, family members, coaches, teachers, ministers, relatives, and others [22,23]. There are no striated social, ethnic, gender, or racial distinctions among traffickers. Often grooming behaviors start with lavish gifts, provision of shelter, offers of fame and a glamorous lifestyle, and promises of a loving relationship. Psychological manipulation often yields to forms of physical control, including threats, financial dependence, fear, substance addiction, and violence [24]. Once victims are targeted and traumatized, complex emotional trauma bonds can be extremely difficult to break. One of the greatest challenges of victim identification is that victims often do not self-identify as such, because the life is normalized [4,12,20,25]. Traffickers can operate in gang-controlled environments, in organized crime rings, or as individuals. The common characteristics of traffickers include their use of force, manipulation, violence, coercion, threats, and/or the creation of psychological and/or physical dependencies to entrench victimization [26]. Contrary to commonly portrayed images of physical bondage of victims, most victims remain tied to their trafficker by invisible tethers, including psychological control and complex trauma bonds, although they also often are manipulated with means of physical control, including beatings and various forms of violence or torture [27]. Often victims feel they are responsible and to blame for poor choices. They may be victims of generational abuse and unaware of their victimization. Victims may feel emotional ties to the only sense of family they have ever known [28]. It is critical for HCPs to understand how HT occurs and develop competencies to aid in trauma-informed victim identification and response [1,29].

ASSESSMENT OF RISK FACTORS

HT has been widely viewed through a criminal justice lens and must be re-framed using a public health model with an upstream approach to rectify health inequities contributing to risk factors and to optimize holistic health impacts arising from a trafficking experience [30,31]. Extensive research efforts have been undertaken to identify risk factors correlating to experiencing LT or child ST [1,2,4,29,32–34]. Although all vulnerable individuals, including children, are at risk for trafficking, disparities in some social determinants of health increase likelihood of encountering opportunity for HT entry (Table 2). An emerging consensus is growing to identify at-risk characteristics of minor victims [12,35]. Recent migration, involvement in the child welfare system, unstable housing, runaway and/or homeless youth, and substance use were identified as the top 5 risk factors for trafficking in reported calls to the National Human Trafficking Resource Center (NHTRC) [5]. These alarming statistics relating to social determinants of health implicate HT as an unparalleled health crisis, with urgent need for informed clinicians to develop and implement effective prevention and intervention strategies. Some risk factors for LT and ST are overlapping, whereas some are distinct.

The landmark pediatric Adverse Childhood Experiences (ACEs) study changed the lens through which clinicians view holistic impacts of trauma across the life span [36]. ACEs include abuse, neglect, and household dysfunction experienced before the age of 18 (Table 3). ACEs have well-established downstream health consequences over the life course. Higher ACEs scores help clinicians predict behavioral health problems in childhood and adulthood, worsening mental health, adverse health-related behaviors, chronic disease

Table 2
Common characteristics among at-risk populations

Labor trafficking	Commercial sex trafficking
Immigrant/migrant status	Homelessness
Debt bondage	Runaway status
Economic disadvantage	Previous placement within foster care, child protective
Low levels of formal education	services, or juvenile justice system(s)
Foreign national status	Substance misuse
Limited employment opportunity	History of abuse, neglect, or exploitation
Questionable employment status	Mental health disorders
Lack of cultural understanding	Family dysfunction, lack of social support
	Identification as lesbian, gay, bisexual, transgender,
	queer, or questioning or intersex
	Physical or mental disability
	Substance misuse or mental illness in family members

Data from Barnert E, Iqbal Z, Bruce J, Anoshiravani A, Kolhatkar G, Greenbaum J. Commercial sexual exploitation and sex trafficking of children and adolescents: a narrative review. Acad Pediatr. 2017; 17(8):825-829 and Roe-Sepowitz D, Bracy K, Lul, B. Arizona State University Office of Sex Trafficking Intervention Research. A four-year analysis of labor trafficking cases in the United States: exploring characteristics and labor trafficking patterns. 2018. Available at: https://socialwork.asu.edu/sites/default/files/stir/v9_national_labor_trafficking_study.pdf.

Table 3 Adverse childhood experiences		
Abuse	**Neglect**	**Household Dysfunction**
Physical	Physical	Mental illness
Emotional	Emotional	Incarcerated relative
Sexual		Mother treated violently
		Substance abuse
		Divorce

Data from Centers for Disease Control and Prevention. About the CDC-Kaiser ACE study. 2019. Available at: https://www.cdc.gov/violenceprevention/childabuseandneglect/acestudy/about.html.

burden, and premature mortality [36]. Because HT encompasses many realms of ACEs classifications, some lessons can be taken from this paradigm and efforts should hone in on prevention to minimize lifelong detrimental consequences. The ACEs study postulates disrupted neurodevelopment after traumatization with subsequent social, emotional, and cognitive impairment that causes a downward cascade of negative health impacts, with risk of early death [12]. Children with a history of sexual abuse (the most reliable predictive factor), in connection with an ACEs score higher than 6 on a scale of 1 to 10, demonstrated increased risk of exploitation by traffickers [29].

HEALTH IMPACTS OF TRAFFICKING

Health impacts are dramatic and multifaceted, including poorly managed chronic medical problems, significant mental health issues, substance abuse/misuse, reproductive or sexual health problems, diminished quality of life, and trauma, while recommended immunizations and other preventive care, including routine dentistry, vaccinations, and health insurance coverage, often are neglected [37]. Victims of HT are considered commodities by traffickers and often are viewed through the lens of economic income earning potential. Health care is not a priority for these victims and typically is accessed when economic profits are in jeopardy with a lack of care or attention to tenets of basic health. There often is failure to comply with follow-up treatment or prescribed therapies [38]. Both LT and ST victims can experience physical trauma and abuse, malnourishment, environmental exposure, and consequences of crowded and/or unsanitary living conditions as well as sleep deprivation and poor nutrition [12]. Victims also may experience depression, suicidality, hopelessness, fearfulness, anxiety, posttraumatic stress disorder (PTSD), lack of affect, disorientation, and substance abuse/misuse or addiction. In particular, for victims of ST, reproductive or sexual complaints are common, including frequent sexually transmitted infections (STIs) and multiple pregnancies and subsequent terminations [30]. Barriers to self-identification or disclosure of victimization include extreme fear, complex trauma bonding, language and/or cultural barriers, lack of identification as victims, and implicit or unconscious bias and/or lack of knowledge of HCPs about HT [39].

PRESENTATION IN THE CLINICAL SETTING

Victim presentation in clinical settings emphasizes the importance of the HCP role [1]. It is important to recognize victims often have been subjected to severe, complex forms of interpersonal trauma that can have an effect on the way they interact with medical professionals [1]. Clinicians should be alert to signs of possible victimization and unfamiliar narratives because individuals often are reluctant to disclose victimization because of guilt, shame, and stigma, meaning these conversations should be skillfully clinician led [1]. Clinicians, however; cannot identify those conditions for which they do not know to look. Lederer and Wetzel [40] found victim presentation in the following clinical environments: (1) emergency departments (63%), (2) outpatient clinics (57%), (3) Planned Parenthood (30%), and primary care clinics (23%). Victims can and do present across the health care continuum, making alertness of the HCP a critical line of defense.

A trauma-informed and victim-centered approach is critical [38,41–43]. Victims have been conditioned to maximize their chance of survival and may tend to elicit negative responses from the HCP. The body language and communication style of patients and those who accompany them should be observed. They may be verbally or physically combative and/or abusive, but these behaviors should be recognized as survival mechanisms [44]. Dignity Health, in partnership with HEAL (Health, Education, Advocacy, Linkage) Trafficking and the Pacific Survivor Center, created the PEARR Tool, a framework for HCPs to employ a trauma-informed approach to victim assistance in the health care setting (Fig. 2) [45]. The PEARR framework consists of (1) providing privacy and using professional interpreters (not patient companions); (2) educating in a nonjudgmental way that normalizes sharing information; (3) allowing time for discussion, including the use of evidence-based tools and asking about identified concerns; and (4) respecting a patient's wishes and responding to safety concerns [45].

All clinicians in all clinical areas should be alert to red flags of a potential trafficking situation presenting for a clinical complaint (Table 4). A provider's first impression of a potential victim may include anxiousness, accompaniment by an overly involved companion; giving false or inconsistent information; appearing confused or disoriented; having no access to identification documents; and possible branding by a trafficker with tattoos [46,47]. It can take weeks, months, or years for victims to self-identify as victims, moving forward to self-identification as "survivor." Often HCPs have unconscious bias affecting belief of victimization [48]. The goal is not to force a patient to disclose his/her trafficking situation and identify as a victim. The goal is to provide a safe space, communicate messages of hope, and facilitate connection to multidisciplinary recovery services, including but not limited to law enforcement, housing, and child protective services. Rescue is not the main objective or responsibility and should not be used as accepted terminology. HCPs can support victims in exiting their trafficking situation [49].

PEARR Tool 🤍 Trauma-Informed Approach to Victim Assistance in Health Care Settings

In partnership with HEAL Trafficking and Pacific Survivor Center, Dignity Health developed this tool, the "PEARR Tool", to guide physicians, social workers, nurses, and other health care professionals on how to provide trauma-informed assistance to patients who are at high risk of abuse, neglect, or violence. The PEARR Tool is based on a universal education approach, which focuses on educating patients about abuse, neglect, or violence prior to, or in lieu of, screening patients with questions.

The goal is to have an informative and normalizing, yet developmentally- and culturally-appropriate, conversation with patients in order to create a context for them to share their own experiences.

A double asterisk [a] indicates points at which this conversation may end. Refer to the double asterisk [a] at the bottom of this page for additional steps. The patient's immediate needs (eg, emergency medical care) should be addressed before use of this tool.

P
Provide Privacy

1. Discuss sensitive topics **alone** and in **safe, private setting** (ideally private room with closed doors). If companion refuses to be separated, then this may be an indicator of abuse, neglect, or violence.[a] Strategies to speak with patient alone: State requirement for private exam or need for patient to be seen alone for radiology, urine test, etc.

   Note: Companions are not appropriate interpreters, regardless of communication abilities. If patient indicates preference to use

companion as interpreter, see your facility's policies for further guidance.[a]

Note: Explain **limits of confidentiality** (i.e., mandated reporting requirements) before beginning any sensitive discussion; however, do not discourage person from disclosing victimization. Patient should feel in control of all disclosures. Mandated reporting includes requirements to report concerns of abuse, neglect, or violence to internal staff and/or to external agencies.

E
Educate

2. Educate patient in manner that is **nonjudgmental** and **normalizes** sharing of information. Example: "I educate all of my patients about [fill in the blank] because violence is so common in our society, and violence has a big impact on our health, safety, and well-being." **Use a brochure or safety card** to review information about abuse, neglect, or violence, and

offer brochure/card to patient. [Ideally, this brochure/card will include information about resources (eg, local service providers, national hotlines)]. Example: "Here are some brochures to take with you in case this is ever an issue for you, **or someone you know.**" If patient declines materials, then respect patient's decision.[a]

A
Ask

3. Allow time for discussion with patient. Example: "Is there anything you'd like to share with me? Do you feel like anyone is hurting your health, safety, or well-being?"[a] If available and when appropriate, use **evidence-based tools** to screen patient for abuse, neglect, or violence.[a]

   Note: All women of reproductive age should be intermittently screened for intimate partner violence (USPSTF Grade B).

4. If there are indicators of victimization, **ASK** about concerns. Example: "I've noticed [insert risk factor/indicator] and I'm concerned for your

health, safety, and well-being. You don't have to share details with me, but I'd like to connect you with resources if you're in need of assistance. Would you like to speak with [insert advocate/service provider]? If not, you can let me know anytime."[a]

Note: **Limit questions** to only those needed to determine patient's safety, to connect patient with resources (eg, trained victim advocates), and to guide your work (eg, perform medical exam).

USPSTF = US Preventive Services Task Force

R R
Respect and Respond

5. If patient denies victimization or declines assistance, then **respect patient's wishes.** If you have **concerns about patient's safety,** offer hotline card or other information about resources that can assist in event of emergency (eg, local shelter, crisis hotline).[a] Otherwise, if patient accepts/requests assistance with accessing services, then **provide personal introduction**

to local victim advocate/service provider; or, **arrange private setting for** patient to call hotline:

National Domestic Violence Hotline, 1-800-799-SAFE (7233);
National Sexual Assault Hotline, 1-800-656-HOPE (4673);
National Human Trafficking Hotline, 1-888-373-7888 [a]

[a] Report **safety concerns** to appropriate staff/departments (eg, nurse supervisor, security). Also, **REPORT** risk factors/indicators as required or permitted by law/regulation, and continue **trauma-informed** health services. Whenever possible, **schedule follow-up appointment** to continue building rapport and to monitor patient's safety/well-being.

Fig. 2. Trauma-informed approach to victim assistance in health care settings. Dignity Health, HEAL Trafficking, Pacific Survivor Center. PEARR Tool: Trauma-Informed Approach to Victim Assistance in Health Care Settings. 2019.

Table 4
Possible red flags for trafficking

Environmental	Emotional/ Psychological	Physical	Cognitive
Poverty	Mental illness	Hunger	Learning disabilities
Recent	Isolation	Malnourishment	Developmental delay
immigration	Emotional distress	Substance misuse/	Lack of formal
status	Family dysfunction	dependency	education
Lack of	History of abuse	Tattoos/branding	Limited English
personal	Depression	Untreated injuries	proficiency
safety	Suicidality	Multiple STIs	
Homelessness	Anxiety	Multiple pregnancy	
Exploitation	PTSD	terminations	
by family	Dissociation	Pregnancy with no	
Lack of social	Lack of affect	prenatal care	
support		Retained foreign bodies	
Foster care		Delayed medical care	
placement		Fatigue	
Juvenile		Dental issues	
justice			
placement			
Abusive			
relationships			

Data from Human Trafficking Hotline. Recognizing the signs. Available at: https://humantraffickinghotline.org/human-trafficking/recognizing-signs. Accessed September 19, 2019.

SCREENING AND DIAGNOSIS

Currently, there is a lack of validated and reliable screening tools, although some preliminary evaluation shows promise for some instruments. Outside directly witnessing abuse or exploitation, a gold standard for diagnosis does not exist [1,50]. Currently, best efforts rely on elevated awareness, clinician intuition, and open-ended questioning with simple, direct questions, examples of which can be found in Table 5. Questions and actions should assess risk of exploitation and/or trafficking, safety, and available services or treatments. *International Classification of Diseases, Tenth Revision (ICD-10)* codes (Table 6) for potential and actual scenarios of both adult and child trafficking were approved in October 2018. These new codes are an effective way to scientifically analyze the number of cases identified and will help aid in understanding the depth of this public health problem. A precautionary aside is to consider that these codes can identify a victim possibly contrary to their wishes and theoretically expose them to potential harm. HCPs may be loath to label an individual, perhaps incorrectly. Careful consideration should be given to mitigating unintended consequences with careful construction of organizational policies surrounding the use of these *ICD-10-CM* codes and their interface with electronic medical records while recognizing the potential benefit to help HT victims across the health care continuum [51].

Table 5
General screening questions for possible victims of human trafficking

Fraud	How did you meet this person/find out about your job?
	What were you told about the job before you started/what promises were made about the relationship? Did your experience meet your expectations?
	Do you feel you were ever deceived about anything related to your job/your relationship?
	Did anything surprise you about this job/relationship?
	Did conditions of your job/relationship change over time?
	Were you ever forced to sign a contract that you did not understand or did not want to sign?
	Did you feel like you understood your rights in this job/situation?
	Did you ever feel like anyone kept you from accessing information about your rights?
Coercion	Did you ever feel pressured to do something that you did not want to do or felt uncomfortable doing?
	What were your expectations of what would happen if you left this person/situation or if you did not do what this person told you to do?
	Did anyone ever take/keep your legal papers or identification for you, such as your passport, visa, driver's license, etc.?
	Did anyone ever threaten you or intimidate you?
	What did this person tell you about what would happen if you were arrested/encountered an immigration official?
	Did you ever see something bad happen to someone else who did not do something that was expected of them? What happened to them? How did that make you feel?
	Did you ever feel that if you left the situation, your life would become more difficult?
Debt	Did you have access to any money/the money you earn? Did anyone take your money or a portion of your money?
	If the money you earned was kept in a bank account, who set up this bank account? Did anyone else beside you have access to the account?
	Were you required to make a certain amount of money every day/week? Why did you feel that you had to meet that amount?
	Did you have fees that you had to pay to someone? How much money did you have left after you paid everything you needed to pay?
	Did you owe any money to anyone in the situation?
	How did you incur this debt? How long have you had the debt?
	Did you feel that it was difficult to pay off your debt? Why?
Force	Did someone control, supervise, or monitor your work/your actions?
	Was your communication ever restricted or monitored?
	Were you able to access medical care?
	Were you ever allowed to leave the place that you were living/working? Under what conditions?
	Was movement outside of your residence/workplace ever monitored or controlled?
	What did you think would have happened if you left the situation?
	Was there ever a time when you wanted to leave but felt that you could not?
	What do you think would have happened if you left without telling anyone?
	Did you feel that it was your only option to stay in the situation?

ST	Did anyone ever pressure you to engage in any sexual acts against your will? Did anyone ever take photos of you and, if so, what did they use them for? Did anyone ever force you to engage in sexual acts with friends or business associates for favors/money? Did anyone ever force you to engage in commercial sex through online Web sites, escort services, street prostitution, informal arrangements, brothels, fake massage businesses, or strip clubs? Were you required to earn a certain amount of money/meet a nightly quota by engaging in commercial sex for someone? What happened if you did not meet this quota? How old were you when you were in this situation? Did you ever see any minors (under 18 years old) involved in commercial sex?
LT	How did you feel about where you worked? How did you feel about your employer/supervisor/crew leader/or other controller? Did you feel that you were paid fairly at this job? What were your normal work hours? How many hours did you have to work each day? What happened if you worked fewer hours or took breaks? Did anyone ever threaten you if you indicated you did not want to work the hours expected of you? Did you have to live in housing provided by the controller? What were the conditions like in this housing?

Data from Polaris Project/National Human trafficking Resource Center. Comprehensive human trafficking assessment. Available at: https://traffickingresourcecenter.org/sites/default/files/Comprehensive%20Trafficking%20Assessment.pdf.

DIFFERENTIAL DIAGNOSIS

Situations of HT share some similarities with intimate partner violence and domestic violence, and, although there can be some overlap, there are significant legal differences and more subtle differences in therapeutic approach. HCPs

Table 6
International Classification of Diseases, Tenth Revision, codes for human trafficking

T74.51	Adult forced sexual exploitation, confirmed
T74.52	Child sexual exploitation, confirmed
T74.61	Adult forced labor exploitation, confirmed
T74.62	Child forced labor exploitation, confirmed
T76.51	Adult forced sexual exploitation, suspected
T76.52	Child sexual exploitation, suspected
T76.61	Adult forced labor exploitation, suspected
T76.62	Child forced labor exploitation, suspected
Y07.6	Multiple perpetrators of maltreatment and neglect
Z04.81	Encounter for examination and observation of victim following forced sexual exploitation
Z04.82	Encounter for examination and observation of victim following forced labor exploitation
Z62.813	Personal history of forced labor or sexual exploitation in childhood
Z91.42	Personal history of forced labor or sexual exploitation

Data from American Hospital Association. ICD-10-CM coding for human trafficking. Available at: https://www.aha.org/icd-10-cm-coding-human-trafficking-resources. Accessed September 21, 2019.

also may miss signs of potential HT by seeing prostitution, drug misuse/addiction, suicidal ideation, and self-harming behaviors through a singular lens without considering a constellation of symptoms suggestive of HT [12].

MANDATORY REPORTING

There is a sensitive line to walk between protecting patient confidentiality and complying with state laws on mandatory reporting, particularly for child victims. If the victim is a minor, state laws governing report of neglect and/or abuse, regardless of whether a child self-identifies as a victim, should be considered carefully and strictly abided by. For adult victims, Health Insurance Portability and Accountability Act (HIPAA) regulations apply, and autonomy of an informed decision-making process should be respected [52]. Clinician consideration for reporting policies should include reporting principles (including sequence and method), documentation, and, most importantly, ensuring compliance with state and federal mandates. HCPs should have a realistic understanding of law enforcement capabilities and limitations along with appraisal of available resources. Clinicians should know some states offer decriminalization or diversion for crimes committed while trafficking whereas others do not, and reporting victims may have implications of criminal charges. Victims should not be viewed or treated as criminals by HCPs, and some states have safe harbor laws to give this protection [52]. There currently is no standardized or uniform response across states, communities, and institutions, although many communities have created multidisciplinary response teams or coalitions, including but not limited to, local police, the Federal Bureau of Investigation, the US Department of Homeland Security, the US Department of Health and Human Services, professional nursing organizations, pro bono legal counsel, faith-based service groups, and advocacy organizations. These groups often collaborate to help victims understand their rights and what specific legal protections and services are available [53].

CLINICIAN MANAGEMENT

Safety is of primary importance for all involved parties, including potential victims, all organizational staff, and other patients and families within the facility. HCPs should establish trust, practice empathetic listening, maintain a nonjudgmental attitude, be open to unfamiliar narratives, offer support, communicate messages of hope, and strive to prevent retraumatization [54]. It is critical to interview patients alone, accomplishing successful separation from both their traffickers and their cell phones. The same words should be used for victims as for patients, and they should not be corrected. For example, victims may call someone an uncle/aunt, family member, or boy/girlfriend when they are not [55,56]. If adult victims are not ready to accept help, their feelings should be validated and normalized. Information on available resources, that they may choose to act on in the future, should be provided discreetly. Health needs should be identified and prioritized, addressing immediate physical needs appropriately within the appropriate scope of practice. HCPs should not proceed as a sexual assault nurse examiner or forensic nurse if they do not have the appropriate education and training to do so. Cultural responsiveness should infuse clinician interactions [57]. If clinicians are ill equipped and unsure and there is no organizational protocol, clinicians should at a minimum call the NHTRC (Fig. 3), while being mindful of HIPAA obligations for adult victims. Trafficking victims present with a higher risk of suicidality, HIV infection, substance misuse, PTSD, STIs, and evidence of violence [1].

ORGANIZATIONAL RESPONSE

There are benefits of implementing an organizational protocol when encountering potential trafficking victims. Key considerations for protocols should include safety precautions, how to handle refusal of care, discharge and multidisciplinary referral considerations, and clinical protocols and/or order sets [12]. Clinical guideline and protocol development should include a robust cadre of disciplines, including clinicians, social workers, administrative staff, and organizational leaders, who assist in policy and procedure development. Multidisciplinary response and development of care models are important for case management, referral, and care coordination [58]. Care should be taken to infuse core principles of a trauma-informed approach, including safety,

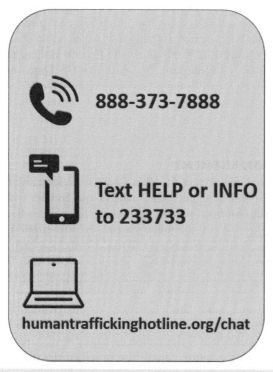

Fig. 3. National Human Trafficking Hotline—24/7.

trustworthiness and transparency, peer support, collaboration, empowerment, humility and responsiveness. Trauma-informed care should not be a checkbox but an evolutionary organizational process. The Missouri Model is a studied comprehensive public health approach that assists in accomplishing culture shifts to view policies, practices, and environments through the lens of trauma [59]. Multidisciplinary resources should consider holistic care, including physical, emotional, psychological, and spiritual care resources. Tangible needs, such as housing, life skills, job training, and procurement of financial income, should be considered along with legal resources and support, addiction treatment, and mental health services.

IMPLICATIONS FOR PRACTICE
Individual clinicians can make a difference by (1) championing the implementation and mandatory use of a protocol within their institutions, (2) learning how to effectively advocate for victims, (3) understanding characteristics of risk and vulnerability, (4) becoming involved with community coalitions or state task forces, and (5) advocating for policies promoting equity in social determinants of health. Clinicians should advocate or participate in conducting rigorous, empirical evaluation research of both intervention and prevention strategies, while advocating for inclusion of multidisciplinary team representatives.

HCPs can work to mobilize an organizational response by (1) working with administrative leadership to implement a multidisciplinary protocol, (2) creating an organizational task force/work group, (3) establishing annual training for all employees, (4) making HT awareness part of onboarding for new staff, (5) working regularly with local/state law enforcement task forces, and (6) encouraging and measuring usage related to *ICD-10* codes on HT.

FNPs and other HCPs can be an effective first responder force by working collectively to raise awareness of HT through evidence-based education, advocating for governmental and institutional policy change, implementing primary prevention measures for identified risk factors, and developing a strong prevention approach with the social-ecological model [1]. Together, HCPs can lead through practice, education, advocacy, and research to promote optimal health outcomes and to end victimization of HT.

Disclosure
The author has nothing to disclose.

References
[1] Greenbaum VJ, Yun K, Todres J. Child trafficking: issues for policies and practice. J Law Med Ethics 2018;46(1):159–63.
[2] Gordon M, Fag S, Coverdale J, et al. Failure to identify a human trafficking victim. Am J Psychiatry 2018;175(5):408–9.
[3] National Institute of Justice. Overview of human trafficking and NIJ's role. 2019. Available at: https://nij.ojp.gov/topics/articles/overview-human-trafficking-and-nijs-role. Accessed September 19, 2019.

[4] Greenbaum J, Bodrick N. Global human trafficking and child victimization. Pediatrics 2017;140(6):1–12.

[5] Polaris. 2018 U.S. national human trafficking hotline statistics. 2018. Available at: https://polarisproject.org/2018-us-national-human-trafficking-hotline-statistics. Accessed September 19, 2019.

[6] Polaris. ABC's American crime. 2019. Available at: https://polarisproject.org/american-crime. Accessed September 19, 2019.

[7] The Joint Commission. Quick safety 42: identifying human trafficking victims. Available at: https://www.jointcommission.org/issues/article.aspx?Article=Dtpt66QSsiI/HRklecKTZ-PAbn6jexdUPHflBjJ/D8Qc=. Accessed September 19, 2019.

[8] International Labour Organization. Forced labour, modern slavery and human trafficking. 2019. Available at: https://www.ilo.org/global/topics/forced-labour/lang--en/index.htm. Accessed September 19, 2019.

[9] United Nations Office on Drugs and Crime. Human trafficking: organized crime and the multibillion dollar sale of people. 2012. Available at: https://www.unodc.org/unodc/en/frontpage/2012/July/human-trafficking_-organized-crime-and-the-multibillion-dollar-sale-of-people.html. Accessed September 19, 2019.

[10] Baldwin SB, Eisenman DP, Sayles JN, et al. Identification of human trafficking victims in health care settings. Health Hum Rights 2011;13(1):E36–49.

[11] Viergever RF, West H, Borland R, et al. Healthcare providers and human trafficking: what do they know, what do they need to know? Findings from the Middle East, the Caribbean, and Central America. Front Public Health 2015;3(6).

[12] Toney-Butler TJ, Mittel O. Human trafficking. Stat Pearls; 2019. Available at: https://www.ncbi.nlm.nih.gov/books/NBK430910/. Accessed September 19, 2019.

[13] Peck JL, Meadows-Oliver M. Human trafficking of children: nurse practitioner knowledge, beliefs, and experience supporting the development of a practice guideline: part one. J Pediatr Health Care 2019;33(5):603–11.

[14] The United States Department of Justice. Key legislation. 2017. Available at: https://www.justice.gov/humantrafficking/key-legislation. Accessed September 19, 2019.

[15] National Human Trafficking Hotline. The action means purpose (AMP) model. 2012. Available at: https://humantraffickinghotline.org/resources/actions-means-purpose-amp-model. Accessed September 19, 2019.

[16] Office on Trafficking in Persons. What is human trafficking?. 2019. Available at: https://www.acf.hhs.gov/otip/about/what-is-human-trafficking. Accessed September 19, 2019.

[17] Shared Hope International. FAQs. 2019. Available at: https://sharedhope.org/the-problem/faqs/. Accessed September 19, 2019.

[18] Miller L. Why labor trafficking is so hard to track. 2019. Available at: https://www.pbs.org/wgbh/frontline/article/why-labor-trafficking-is-so-hard-to-track/. Accessed September 19, 2019.

[19] Unicef. What fuels human trafficking?. 2017. Available at: https://www.unicefusa.org/stories/what-fuels-human-trafficking/31692. Accessed September 19, 2019.

[20] Data from the American Hospital Association. Dispelling myths about human trafficking for health care providers. 2018. Available at: https://www.aha.org/news/insights-and-analysis/2018-01-05-dispelling-myths-about-human-trafficking-health-care. Accessed September 19, 2019.

[21] National Human Trafficking Hotline. The traffickers. 2019. Available at: https://humantraffickinghotline.org/what-human-trafficking/human-trafficking/traffickers. Accessed September 19, 2019.

[22] Recknor FH. Health-care provider challenges to the identification of human trafficking in health-care settings: a qualitative study. J Hum Traffick 2018;4(3):213–30.

[23] McCain Institute. A six-year analysis of sex traffickers of minors. Available at: https://www.mccaininstitute.org/six-year-analysis-of-sex-traffickers/. Accessed September 19, 2019.

[24] Polaris. The victims & traffickers. 2019. Available at: https://polarisproject.org/victims-traffickers. Accessed September 19, 2019.

[25] Office for Victims of Crime. Understanding human trafficking. 2019. Available at: https://www.ovcttac.gov/taskforceguide/eguide/1-understanding-human-trafficking/. Accessed September 19, 2019.

[26] Deshpande N, Nour NM. Sex trafficking of women and girls. Rev Obstet Gynecol 2013;6(10):e22–7.

[27] Macy RJ, Graham LM. Identifying domestic and international sex-trafficking victims during human service provision. Trauma Violence Abuse 2012;13(2):59–76.

[28] Ohio Justice and Policy Center. The power of blame. Available at: http://www.ohiojpc.org/the-power-of-blame/. Accessed September 19, 2019.

[29] Reid JA, Baglivio M, Piquero AR, et al. Human trafficking of minors and childhood adversity in Florida. Am J Public Health 2017;107(2):306–11.

[30] Greenbaum J. Introduction to human trafficking: who is affected?. In: Chisolm-Straker M, Stoklosa H, editors. Human trafficking is a public health issue: a paradigm expansion in the United States. Cham (Switzerland): Springer; 2017. p. 1–14.

[31] Centers for Disease Control and Prevention. Violence prevention: the social-ecological model. Available at: https://www.cdc.gov/violenceprevention/publichealthissue/social-ecologicalmodel.html. Accessed September 19, 2019.

[32] Gibbs DA, Henninger AM, Tueller SJ, et al. Human trafficking and the child welfare population in Florida. Child Youth Serv Rev 2018;88(2018):1–10.

[33] Goldberg AP, Moore JL, Houck C, et al. Domestic minor sex trafficking patients: a retrospective analysis of medial presentation. J Pediatr Adolesc Gynecol 2016;30(2017):109–15.

[34] Havlicek J, Huston S, Boughton S, et al. Human trafficking of children in Illinois: prevalence and characteristics. Child Youth Serv Rev 2016;69(2016):127–35.

[35] Rothma EF, Stoklosa H, Baldwin SB, et al. HEAL Trafficking. Public health research priorities to address US human trafficking. Am J Public Health 2017;107(7):1045–7.

[36] Centers for Disease Control and Prevention. About the CDC-Kaiser ACE study. 2019. Available at: https://www.cdc.gov/violenceprevention/childabuseandneglect/acestudy/about.html. Accessed September 19, 2019.

[37] Department of Health and Human Services. Resources: common health issues seen in victims of human trafficking. Available at: https://www.acf.hhs.goc>orr>health_problems_seen_in_traffick_victims.html. Accessed September 19, 2019.

[38] Macias-Konstantopoulos WM. Caring for the trafficked patient: ethical challenges and recommendations for health care professionals. AMA J Ethics 2017;19(1):80–90.

[39] Hopper EK, Gonzales LD. A comparison of psychological symptoms in survivors of sex and labor trafficking. Behav Med 2018;44(3):177–88.

[40] Lederer LJ, Wetzel CA. The health consequences of sex trafficking and their implications for identifying victims in healthcare facilities. Ann Health Law 2014;23(1):61.

[41] Hopper E. Trauma-informed psychological assessment of human trafficking survivors. Women Ther 2016;40(1–2):12–30.

[42] Rollins R, Gribble A, Barrett SE, et al. Who is in your waiting room? Health care professionals as culturally responsive and trauma-informed first responders to human trafficking. AMA J Ethics 2017;19(1):63–71. Available at: https://journalofethics.ama-assn.org/article/who-your-waiting-room-health-care-professionals-culturally-responsive-and-trauma-informed-first/2017-01. Accessed September 19, 2019.

[43] Office for Victims of Crime Training and Technical Assistance Center. Using a trauma-informed approach. Available at: https://www.ovcttac.gov/taskforceguide/eguide/4-supporting-victims/41-using-a-trauma-informed-approach/. Accessed September 19, 2019.

[44] Judge AM, Murphy JA, Hidalgo J, et al. Engaging survivors of human trafficking: complex health care needs and scarce resources. Ann Intern Med 2018;168(9):658–63.

[45] Dignity Health. Using the PEARR tool. Available at: https://www.dignityhealth.org/hello-humankindness/human-trafficking/victim-centered-and-trauma-informed/using-the-pearr-tool. Accessed September 19, 2019.

[46] Polaris. Recognize the signs. Available at: https://polarisproject.org/human-trafficking/recognize-signs. Accessed September 19, 2019.

[47] NAPNAP Partners for Vulnerable Youth. Tattoos of human trafficking victims. Available at: https://www.napnappartners.org/tattoos-human-trafficking-victims. Accessed September 19, 2019.

[48] Cunningham KC, DeMarni-Cromer L. Attitudes about human trafficking: individual differences related to belief and victim blame. J Interpers Violence 2016;31(2):228–44.

[49] Institute of Medicine and National Research Council. Confronting commercial sexual exploitation and sex trafficking of minors in the United States: a guide for the health care sector. Available at: https://www.nap.edu/read/18886/chapter/4. Accessed September 19, 2019.

[50] Greenbaum VJ, Livings LS, Lai BS, et al. Evaluation of a tool to identify child sex trafficking victims in multiple healthcare settings. J Adolesc Health 2018;63(6):745–52.

[51] Greenbaum J, Stoklosa H. The healthcare response to human trafficking: a need for globally harmonized ICD codes. PLoS Med 2019;16(5):e1002799.

[52] English A. Mandatory reporting of human trafficking: potential benefits and risks of harm. AMA J Ethics 2017;19(1):54–62.

[53] Office for Victims of Crime Training and Technical Assistance Center. Human trafficking task force e-guide. Available at: https://www.ovcttac.gov/taskforceguide/eguide/. Accessed September 19, 2019.

[54] Dovydaitis T. Human trafficking: the role of the health care provider. J Midwifery Womens Health 2011;55(5):462–7.

[55] Even E, Dateline @ TJC. Identifying human trafficking victims among your patients. 2017. Available at: https://www.jointcommission.org/dateline_tjc/identifying_human_trafficking_victims_among_your_patients/. Accessed September 19, 2019.

[56] National Conference of State Legislatures. Human trafficking and the health care system. 2019. Available at: http://www.ncsl.org/research/health/human-trafficking-and-the-health-care-system.aspx. Accessed September 19, 2019.

[57] Cheshire WP. Groupthink: how should clinicians respond to human trafficking? AMA J Ethics 2017;17(1):91–7.

[58] Stoklosa H, Grace AM, Littenberg N. Medical education on human trafficking. AMA J Ethics 2015;l17(10):914–21.

[59] Missouri Department of Mental Health. Trauma informed care. Available at: https://dmh.mo.gov/trauma/. Accessed September 19, 2019.

Advances in Family Practice Nursing 2 (2020) 187–199

ADVANCES IN FAMILY PRACTICE NURSING

Pediatric Fecal Incontinence Evaluation and Management in Primary Care

Mary Lauren Pfieffer, DNP, FNP-BC, CPN*

Vanderbilt University School of Nursing, Nashville, TN, USA

Keywords

- Encopresis • Soiling • Fecal incontinence (FI)
- Functional nonretentive fecal incontinence (FNRFI)
- Nonretentive fecal incontinence (NFI) • Bowel dysfunction
- Functional constipation

Key points

- Pediatric fecal incontinence (FI) is related to either functional constipation or functional nonretentive fecal incontinence (FNRFI). It is important to differentiate as it influences treatment.

- History for FI includes thorough bowel movement history with incontinence characteristics, dietary history, behavioral history, coinciding urinary concerns, and any other health complaints.

- Health care providers should complete a thorough physical examination for suspected FI, focusing on gastrointestinal, genitourinary, neurologic, lower musculoskeletal and psychiatric systems, and a rectal examination.

- After initial impaction is cleared, treatment is a blend of pharmacologic and nonpharmacological approaches focusing on enhanced toilet training and maintenance laxatives.

- Follow-up by health care providers is vital, as FI can be a long-term condition and relapse of symptoms occurs frequently.

INTRODUCTION

Fecal incontinence (FI) is a multifactorial diagnosis related to the involuntary passage of feces, not related to underlying illness, after bowel continence is obtained. This is diagnosed after age 4, which is the age bowel continence is

*461 21st Avenue South, Frist Hall 354, Nashville, TN 37240. E-mail address: mary.pfieffer@vanderbilt.edu

https://doi.org/10.1016/j.yfpn.2020.01.007
2589-420X/20/

expected in children [1]. FI, functional nonretentive fecal incontinence (FNRFI), nonretentive fecal incontinence (NFI), encopresis, and soiling are terms that are used interchangeably; however, FI and FNRFI are the preferred terms [2,3]. Historically there have been primary and secondary encopresis and these terms are still seen in literature. Primary encopresis occurs when patient has never been toilet trained, and secondary encopresis occurs when patient was toilet trained and experiences subsequent FI [4]. The prevalence of FI is 3% to 7% worldwide and occurs more often in male than female individuals [5–7]. Research show ratios are 6:1 and sometimes 3:1 among male to female patients [5,6]. FI occurs more frequently in urban areas and in patients of lower socioeconomic backgrounds [6].

It is important to differentiate delayed toilet training and delayed bowel training from FI. Patients with FI often unintentionally leak unformed stool into underwear but also will often use toilet to pass stool if able [1], whereas patients with delayed bowel training withhold stool and refuse to use toilet [8]. Patients with delayed bowel training have normal formed bowel movements in diaper or pull-up but refuse toileting most often related to fear and anxiety of the toilet or the passage of the stool [1].

HISTORY

Eighty percent of patients with FI have functional constipation [3,8]. Generally, patients with functional constipation unintentionally develop FI and pass liquid or soft stool into underwear. It is important to know if the patient is constipated, as it will determine treatment plan. Patients with FNRFI have FI but do not have constipation or fecal retention of stool [3].

There are several risk factors for FI. Providers need to perform a dietary recall, as patients who consume low-fiber diets are at risk for FI related to constipation risk [4]. Also, pediatric growth charts can identify if FI led to any growth restrictions [1]. Certain medications cause constipation and therefore increase risk of FI. Last, psychological diagnoses, such as anxiety and depression, autism spectrum disorder, and/or attention-deficit disorder/attention-deficit/hyperactivity disorder (ADD/ADHD) increase risk of encopresis [7,9]. Research shows that 30% to 50% of patients with FI have additional behavioral or psychiatric disorder [9]. Children with ADD/ADHD are extremely distracted to conclude activity and have a bowel movement [7]. There is also an increased likelihood of FI if a patient has been sexually assaulted [10].

Patients with FI may present with abdominal pain, decreased appetite, enuresis, passage of stools that have a tendency to clog the toilet, and/or constipation. Patients often will report painful passage of stool, which results in stool withholding and this leads to constipation [7]. Most patients with FI present with involuntary leakage of stool into underwear. FI is an emotionally distressing complaint for patient and caregiver. FI can negatively impact quality of life. It can lead to guilt and shame and carry lifelong consequences for the patient and family [11].

Providers need to request a thorough bowel habit history. Providers should have a copy of the Bristol stool form scale in clinic. This will help streamline stool language and description [1,12]. How many times a week is FI occurring? Can the child sense the need to have a bowel movement? If the patient cannot feel need to defecate, neurologic dysfunction may be present [7]. What is the consistency of stool leaked (solid/hard, liquid, semiformed, thin and ribbon-like)? If stools are thin and ribbonlike, Hirschsprung disease should be suspected. Did it hurt to pass stool? Did the stool clog the toilet? Providers should suspect FI stemming from constipation if stool clogs the toilet [13]. Did the patient have to strain to pass stool? What time of day is stool leaked? Some older children with FI are able to hold any stool for when they are home in later afternoons or evenings [3]. Passing stool at home can help decrease patient anxiety surrounding inconsistent stool patterns and having to pass it in a public place.

FI can also coincide with urinary incontinence (UI), therefore genitourinary history questions are essential [3]. How often is UI occurring? Does UI only happen at night? How often does the patient void? What is typical liquid consumption pattern? Any urinary tract infection symptoms? A urinary tract infection could also complicate FI [14].

CASE STUDY

Tommy is an 8-year-old boy who presents to the clinic with his mom complaining of stool leakage and trouble defecating. This has been going on for the past 6 months with no resolution with interventions at home.

History

He was toilet trained with no issues at 3.5 year old. He started passing small amounts of liquid stool into underwear 3 times a week approximately 6 months ago. Tommy initially felt constipated but does not feel that currently. He has some abdominal pain and reports pain with defecation. The toilet bowl generally gets clogged when he is able to have a bowel movement. He usually has to spend an hour in bathroom to pass his stool. This occurs about once every 2 weeks. No blood is noted by the patient or his mom. The patient and his mom deny urinary symptoms. His diet is high in carbohydrates. He does not like fruits or vegetables and his mom describes him as a picky eater and he often has a lack of appetite. Tommy has followed typical growth and development patterns. He was diagnosed with ADHD last year after performing poorly in school and he was put on methylphenidate (Quillivant XR) for management. He is in the third grade and performing well this year. He is on no other medications. Socially he lives at home with mom and younger sister. His dad is an alcoholic and Tommy has no contact with him. Both patient and mom are visibly distressed regarding this situation.

His physical examination is noted to be mostly normal. There is some distention of abdomen noted. There is also decrease bowel sounds in lower quadrants. Genitourinary examination is normal. Neurologic examination is normal. Musculoskeletal examination is normal. Psychiatric examination is not revealing. The patient is not withdrawn or fidgety. He is open to discussing his symptoms, as he is wanting a resolution. Digital rectal examination (DRE) reveals normal sphincter tone but fecal mass is present. Perianal irritation is noted. Stool leakage is noted on underwear.

Diagnostics and diagnosis

As functional constipation is suspected to be causing Tommy's FI, there were not many diagnostics ordered, much to the dismay of the family. They were willing to undergo testing to increase chances of swifter symptom resolution. Thyroid laboratory tests and celiac testing were negative. Psychosocial and behavioral screenings were negative. Abdominal radiograph was revealing of a large amount of stool in the colon. Tommy has not evacuated stool completely in 10 days. No other diagnostics were ordered, as they would not change treatment pattern. The patient meets criteria for functional constipation FI based on the ROME IV criteria. He has had FI at least once a week for 1 month. He has had consistent symptoms for 6 months and other differentials have been ruled out.

ASSESSMENT

It is essential to do a thorough physical examination with suspected FI. The systems that will need to be focused on are gastrointestinal (GI), genitourinary, neurologic, lower musculoskeletal, psychiatric, and rectal examinations. The GI portion of the assessment will focus on abdominal inspection, palpation, and auscultation. It is important to inspect the abdomen to see if it is distended. Also observe if the patient appears uncomfortable related to retention of fecal matter. Next, the provider should progress to light and deep abdominal palpation. Tenderness to palpation could strengthen constipation differential [1]. If a patient has decreased or absent bowel sounds with auscultation, constipation is suspected.

A genitourinary examination would be short but necessary, as anatomic abnormalities may predispose the patient to urinary incontinence or FI [14]. Providers need to assess for labial irritations or adhesions, meatal abnormalities, and/or glandular irritation, as these findings can be revealing for urinary or fecal incontinence causes [14]. Understandably, assessment for sexual abuse also should be evaluated during the genitourinary examination [14].

A neurologic examination for FI would typically include assessment of the lower half of the body. Additional assessment and diagnostics would be necessary if there were abnormals appreciated in lower extremity muscle tone, lower extremity deep tendon reflexes, and lower extremity strength [1]. Muscle weakness or atrophy of lower extremities also could lead to urinary tract infections, which could lead to FI [14].

A musculoskeletal examination would be looking primarily at the spine to identify conditions involving the spinal dysraphism [15]. Providers need to inspect the gluteal cleft and perform spinal range of motion. Gluteal cleft deviation is related to asymmetry, and this is an abnormal finding [15]. A sacral dimple or spinal abnormalities would require further investigation [1]. Corresponding spinal abnormalities could lead to functional stool pattern problems and increase risk for FI [15].

Observation during examinations lend many providers answers to psychiatric concerns. Is the child fidgety and unable to sit still during the examination? ADD/ADHD may need to be evaluated. Do patients appear withdrawn during examination? Then abuse may be suspected. Are they embarrassed to talk about toileting? Always remember how emotionally distressing this can be for patients and families, as patients know FI is not a social norm and they should have bowel movements in the toilet. Providers also need to observe for bowel delaying tactics. The Vincent curtsey is often seen with bladder incontinence, but also can be seen with bowel incontinence [14]. This is where patient bends down at the waist while crossing ones' legs [14]. Often patients with FI will not want to squat, as this will increase urge to defecate [1].

Last, a rectal examination is often performed. It is not an examination performed without careful consideration if it would change treatment. A DRE can be very distressing to a child, especially if there is a past history of abuse or there has been pain with passage of the stool [1,15]. Abuse would be suspected if the patient has a large, dilated rectum with scaring or bruising [15]. Providers could observe for fissures, hemorrhoids, displacement of rectum, and fecal matter with inspection of the rectum [1]. Anal fissures or hemorrhoids show that stool passage is painful for the patient related to large-diameter stools [3]. Observing fecal matter around the rectum, underwear, or diaper can help providers discern the category on the Bristol stool scale. A DRE examination would assess for rectal masses, fecal stool mass, sphincter tone, and stool composition [1,15]. Some patients have perianal skin irritation related to this leakage of stool [15].

PATHOPHYSIOLOGY

Bowel movement production involves the external and internal anal sphincter, rectal muscles, and rectum [1]. Naturally ceased the internal and external anal sphincters are contracted and this prohibits fecal incontinence [1]. An individual will feel the need to defecate when the stool hits the rectal wall. When an individual does not relax sphincters and allow stool to evacuate, the stool is pushed back into the rectum and fecal load increases [1]. This cycle creates dilation and extension of the rectum and a formation of a large fecal mass. Consequently, FI occurs as stool continues to be pushed into the rectum, causing loose, liquid stool to be pushed around the hard fecal mass [4]. Fissures and hemorrhoids are causes for initial fecal withholding, as patients do not want to experience pain with defecation. Rectal prolapse is a potential for patients with FI when trying to defecate around this fecal mass [1]. Patients who have chronic constipation are at risk for FI related to chronic stretching of the rectum from constipation.

The bowel and bladder systems are often correlated. Stretching of the rectum can pose problems for the bladder. Likewise, conditions related to bladder filling influence anorectal pressure and anorectal sensation [16]. Rectal distention similarly causes bladder dysfunction, especially issues with bladder sensation and bladder capacity [16]. More studies are needed to support the bladder and bowel interrelation findings.

DIAGNOSIS

Rome IV criteria are used when making clinical diagnosis for functional constipation related to FI and FNRFI [2]. These diagnoses necessitate evaluation to rule out other differentials [2]. Rome III to Rome IV decreased symptom length from 2 months to 1 month [2]. Both require the child to be 4 years old (developmentally and numerically) [2].

Diagnosis of functional constipation requires 2 or more of the following that occur at least once per week for 1 month [2]:

- Greater than or equal to 2 defecations in toilet per week
- FI once a week
- Stool retention
- Painful or hard stools
- Fecal mass presence
- History of toilet obstruction from stool evacuation

Diagnosis of FNRFI requires 1-month history of the following [2]:

- No fecal retention or fecal mass
- Inappropriate defecation locations
- Thorough evaluation to rule out other FI differentials

DIFFERENTIAL DIAGNOSIS

- Anal atresia [1,5,7,8]
- Anal fissure
- Anal fistula
- Anal trauma or abuse
- Endocrine causes (hypothyroidism, hypercalcemia)
- Functional constipation
- Hirschsprung disease
- Hypothyroidism/hypoparathyroidism
- Hypotonia causes (eg, cerebral palsy)
- Inflammatory bowel disorder (ulcerative colitis, Crohn's disease)
- Medication use (narcotics containing codeine, antacids)
- Pelvic floor dysfunction
- Spinal cord disorder or tumor

DIAGNOSTIC TESTING

Some diagnostic tests could be clinically indicated, although not always necessary: laboratory tests, radiographs, colonic transit times (CTTs), rectal biopsy, and anorectal manometry. Laboratory tests are often not necessary, but if doing thyroid laboratory tests, celiac testing and electrolytes (including calcium and magnesium) would be appropriate [1]. Magnesium levels could indicate laxative abuse [7]. Allergy testing could reveal cow milk protein allergy [1].

Radiographs help to identify if there are abnormalities within the abdomen or spine that could complicate FI. Abdominal radiographs allow visualization of how much stool is in the colon [1]. There is some controversy surrounding the sensitivity and specificity of abdominal radiographs, but some clinicians argue that these are relatively inexpensive, and it will clearly show parents and patients a picture of stool buildup [15]. Palpating a fecal mass with DRE is sufficient to prove FI, but in some patients, it is impossible to examine (obese and sexual abuse cases), and abdominal radiographs could aid diagnosis [15]. Some clinicians order barium enemas in this clinical scenario. This test gives information regarding the colon and rules out colonic obstruction [1]. Barium enemas also can rule out Hirschsprung disease [7]. Lumbosacral radiographs should be performed only if spine/lower extremity examination is abnormal [7].

CTTs are evaluated when constipation is questioned [3,15]. CTT looks at transit time of the stool in the intestines. CTT is decreased in those who are constipated [2]. Performing this test can differentiate functional constipation and FNRFI, and it can then change treatment trajectory [15]. Roughly 50% of patients with a delayed CTT are constipated [15]. A normal CTT is seen 90% of the time in patients with FNRFI [15].

Rectal biopsies are clinically indicated if Hirschsprung disease is suspected [1]. These are mostly performed in infants [1]. This can be performed under anesthesia or with a rectal suction biopsy. Hirschsprung disease would be confirmed if there was an absence of ganglion cells [1,7]. Anorectal manometry is necessary to confirm a negative result if Hirschsprung disease is suspected but rectal biopsy is negative.

Anorectal manometry is a highly specialized test that looks at anorectal sensorimotor function and sphincter tone [15]. It also assesses rectal sensation and rectoanal inhibitory reflex [1,15]. Hirschsprung disease can further be ruled out of differentials if there is normal internal rectal sphincter tone and normal rectal dilation with colon transit [1]. Patients with FNRFI often have normal sensation and anal sphincter tone but abnormal defecation dynamics [15].

Other miscellaneous tests that could be considered include abdominal ultrasound and rectal barostat. Abdominal ultrasounds are not clinically indicated in a patient with FI. There is evidence to support their use in evaluating rectal diameter and fecal impaction, but is not necessary for diagnosis [15]. There is hope that abdominal ultrasounds can decrease the need for DRE in the future [3]. A rectal barostat is also discussed in the literature as a way to assess anorectal function and rectal compliance [15]. There are no clinical findings to support routine use in patients [3,15].

TREATMENT

The treatment of FI is multimodal and requires nonpharmacological and pharmacologic intervention [3]. Health care providers need to treat underlying conditions or diseases if present. Plan of care for patients with constipation is to undergo initial bowel cleanout and then establish a regular bowel habit pattern. Plan of care for patients with FNRFI is behavioral therapy and establishing regular bowel habits.

Nonpharmacologic

Education regarding constipation and the details regarding defecation is paramount for FI and FNRFI treatment [1,17]. The literature speaks immensely regarding enhanced toilet training (ETT). ETT is behavioral therapy that helps establish regular bowel habits for patients [1,17,18]. Patients should have regular sitting time on the toilet, preferably after meals, to maximize use of the gastrocolic reflex [1]. Literature differs on time needed to sit on the toilet for effectiveness, but anywhere from 5 to 30 minutes is appropriate [1,15]. ETT also includes patient education regarding muscle straining and muscle relaxing that occurs with defecation [18]. ETT needs to occur in a stress-free and peaceful environment [15]. Breathing techniques around defecation also need to be discussed, as general fear around defecation can cause breath-holding. A reward system generally is effective in this training [1,15]. Starting with rewarding for being in the room with the toilet is appropriate, with the end goal to be defecation into the toilet [1]. ETT should begin the same time as pharmacologic interventions to maintain success of pharmacologic intervention [1]. ETT significantly decreases FI and FNRFI episodes in patients and decreases need for other treatments [18].

Frequently, patients with FI need counseling to help with psychosocial issues surrounding bowel leakage. Sexual abuse victims will need appropriate psychological treatment [2]. Quality of life is impacted in patients with FI and FNRFI, as they feel humiliation, embarrassment, and responsible for this condition [15]. Referral to counselors is important for parents of patients with FI and FNRFI, as they can experience the same emotional turmoil [15]. Parents often feel the patient is purposefully having FI and they need to be educated that this is not accurate [17]. The prevalence of other behavioral conditions is high in those who have FI, and longevity of treatments is another encourager for patient and parental counseling [1].

Improving dietary intake can be helpful for patients with FI or FNRFI. Health care providers will often encourage patients to increase fluid intake, increase fiber, decrease dairy, and initiate a probiotic to combat constipation. Increasing fluid intake can help with constipation only if the patient is dehydrated [17]. Children generally do not consume enough nondairy beverages, so encouraging water intake is an appropriate intervention. Data are mixed related to increasing fiber-rich foods to help FI [1,19]. Increasing fiber can either make stool softer and easier to pass or it can increase size of stool, causing distension of rectum and greater impaction [17]. Health care providers should encourage fiber at a calculated level by the child's age plus 5 to 10 g per day for patients with mild constipation [17]. Dairy has mixed effects on patients' bowel habits. Dairy can increase constipation and bowel problems if there is an intolerance to milk protein. Patients who have atopy have an increased chance of having a milk protein intolerance or allergy [17]. Many studies suggest a trial off dairy for 2 weeks to see if there is an improvement in symptoms [19]. Initiating a prebiotic or probiotic has also been seen in the literature as an intervention for constipation [20]. These supplements decrease CTT, increase bowel movement frequency, and decrease constipation-associated discomfort [1]. Currently, there are not enough data to support this intervention [1,19].

Biofeedback technique is used to educate patients regarding anal sphincter muscles [18]. Placing electrodes around the anus assists in tightening and relaxing muscles [18]. This is used only in conjunction with ETT and pharmacologic management. This is not useful for all patients. Some studies show biofeedback is not any more effective than laxatives [17].

Pharmacologic

The initial disimpaction for a patient with constipation-related FI will include laxatives and enemas if treated outpatient, or nasogastric polyethylene glycol solution if treated inpatient [1,15]. A lubricant can be used around the anus to help with bowel passage if the patient has anal fissures. Laxatives are not recommended for patients with FNRFI, as it will make patients have a difficult time retaining stool [3,15]. There are some off-label medications that can be used in patients who have FNRFI if behavioral therapy and ETT are not effective.

Laxatives have a role in treating patients with FI who are constipated or are impacted. If impaction is present, removal of that impaction is necessary to allow the patient to begin a normal stool pattern [1]. Removal of impaction can be achieved by laxative use, enemas, and/or manual disimpaction in the outpatient setting [1]. Polyethylene glycol solution (such as MiraLAX) is indicated first-line for treatment [2,19]. It is prescribed 1.0 to 1.5 g per kilogram per day by mouth for up to 6 days [17]. It is difficult to get pediatric patients to take this volume by mouth, therefore parental encouragement is essential. Inpatient treatment of nasogastric polyethylene glycol-electrolyte solution, such as Go-LYTELY, would be recommended for initial disimpaction if unable to take that volume by mouth. Mineral oil is a lubricant laxative and is indicated for initial disimpaction for patients with FI with constipation. The recommended dose is 15 to 30 mL per year of age by mouth, with the maximum intake of 240 mL per day [17]. This should be prescribed only in those who do not have a risk for aspiration, as it can cause a lipoid pneumonia if aspirated [17].

After initial bowel disimpaction is completed, laxatives continue to have a place in treatment of patients with FI [1,17]. The goal is for patients to have 1 to 2 soft stools a day, and laxative use can help achieve that. Laxatives used for maintenance for patients with FI are polyethylene glycol solution (MiraLAX), magnesium hydroxide (milk of magnesia), lactulose, and mineral oil

[1,17]. Polyethylene glycol solution (such as MiraLAX) is recommended at 0.4 to 0.8 g per kilogram per day (maximum is 17 g per day) [17]. Potential side effects seen with polyethylene glycol are diarrhea, bloating, and/or abdominal pain [1,17]. Magnesium hydroxide (milk of magnesia) is an osmotic laxative that increases gastric motility [17]. It is recommended at a 1 to 3 mL per kilogram daily dose to maintain soft stools [1,17]. A potential side effect is hypermagnesemia, so use caution when prescribing to certain populations. Lactulose is another osmotic laxative used for treatment of constipation-related FI. It is recommended at a 1 mL per kilogram (up to 30 mL) dosage given once or twice daily [1,17]. Side effects of lactulose are gassiness and abdominal cramping [17]. Mineral oil can be prescribed 1 to 3 mL per kilogram daily to maintain soft stools [17]. This medication lubricates the intestine and reduces water absorption into the intestine [1]. The caution with aspiration remains the same with this dosage as well. Bisacodyl (Dulcolax) is also an option for treatment, but health care providers are encouraged to use this only in patients of adolescent age or older [17]. It is a stimulant laxative and can be given by mouth or rectally as a suppository. The dosing is the same regardless of route. Patients 3 to 10 years of age will take 5 mg per day and patients older than 10 years will take 5 to 10 mg per day [3]. This medication needs to be taken at night, as when taken orally it can take approximately 6 hours to work [3]. Side effects with this medication are diarrhea, nausea, and abdominal pain [3].

Enemas and suppositories are generally only used for treatment of initial fecal impaction. Sodium docusate enema has been shown to have equal effectiveness with removal of initial impaction as polyethylene glycol solution [21]. It is given to patients younger than 6 years at a dose of 60 mL, and for patients older than 6 years at a dose of 120 mL [3]. Other enemas that could be used are sodium phosphate enemas, saline enemas, and mineral oil enemas [3,17]. Oral treatment is the indicated first-line treatment for FI, as patients have a negative experience with defecation [1].

Antianxiety and antidepressants are appropriate in some patients with FI and FNRFI. These medications should be prescribed only if there is an appropriate diagnosis associated with the patient [3]. Antianxiety and antidepressants are not indicated for FI and FNRFI but rather for the anxiety or depression that could be causing the incontinence. The medications most often prescribed in the pediatric population are selective serotonin reuptake inhibitors [3].

Patients with FNRFI can be prescribed off-label loperamide or imipramine [3,15]. Loperamide is approved to treat diarrhea but not FNRFI. It works to stop peristalsis and increases CTT [22]. It also improves anal sphincter tone, decreasing stool leakage [15]. Health care providers need to be cautious with prescribing loperamide as the Food and Drug Administration has put out a warning for potential cardiac and abuse effects [23]. Imipramine is a nontricyclic antidepressant that has anticholinergic effects on patients. These anticholinergic effects have been seen to delay gastric motility and improve anal sphincter tone [15]. It has been prescribed off label for some patients with FNRFI. There is a black box warning for increased suicidality (especially in the pediatric population) and potential cardiovascular effects with this medication, so caution with prescribing is encouraged [15].

REFERRALS AND FOLLOW-UP

Most patients with FI and FNRFI can be treated within primary care. Patient may need to see GI, neurology, or psychiatric specialists if there are associated comorbidities. If FI is untreated, it can lead to comorbidities, such as "enuresis, frequent urinary tract infections, rectal prolapse, or pelvic dyssynergia" [1] (p394). A GI provider or general surgeon would do manual removal of fecal impaction, as this is often done under general anesthesia to decrease trauma to the patient [1]. Patients need close observation with initial bowel cleanout and seen every 3 or 4 days afterward to evaluate effectiveness [17]. Providers also need to ensure that removal of fecal impaction is not necessary [17]. Patients should be seen at least monthly after initial bowel cleanout to ensure that bowel regimen, laxative dosing titration, and behavioral therapies are appropriate [17].

Children treated for FI and FNRFI may not feel the urge to eliminate stool for upward of a year, so supporting families through this diagnosis is important. The shorter duration of symptoms is related to a faster recovery. Recovery rates for FI are roughly 30% to 50% at 1 year and 48% to 75% after 5 years [8,17]. Recovery rates for FNRFI are much lower, as after 2 years of treatment, only 29% were cured [3,15]. Relapse occurs often for both FI and FNRFI, therefore close follow-up is paramount for treatment success.

SUMMARY

FI is seen frequently in primary care. It is related to the involuntary passage of feces after developmentally appropriate bowel continence is obtained. It is associated with functional constipation or FNRFI. Management depends on the presenting symptoms but begins with disimpaction if necessary. Then treatment includes a blend of nonpharmacologic ETT and behavioral therapy and pharmacologic laxatives. Close follow-up is paramount, as this is a long-term condition and relapse of symptoms frequently happens. Ensuring the patient is educated is important and may help improve long-term quality of life for the patient.

CASE CONCLUSION

Tommy's initial cleanout plan included polyethylene glycol solution (Mira-LAX) dosed at 1.0 to 1.5 g per kilogram per day by mouth for 6 days. Patient education was given to the patient and family regarding ETT, and the patient was encouraged to have timed toilet sitting after meals and before bed anywhere from 5 to 30 minutes in length. After initial cleanout and physical examination has been completed to ensure that the fecal mass is out, maintenance polyethylene glycol solution is prescribed to Tommy at a dosage of 0.4 to 0.8 g per kilogram per day (maximum is 17 g per day). The health care provider also encouraged increase in fluids and fiber and an added probiotic.

Referral was given to counseling for both parents and the patient to support this challenging diagnosis.

Tommy and his family were seen frequently at the beginning of treatment: every 3 days for 2 weeks and then every 2 weeks for 2 months to ensure that bowel frequency was appropriate and to applaud successes. Subsequently, follow-up timing decreased to every 2 months for the next year. As time went on, maintenance polyethylene glycol solution compliance decreased and FI symptoms reemerged and Tommy and his family were back at the clinic. Initial treatment was restarted. Psychosocial and behavioral screenings were indicative of anxiety at this visit. Thirty percent to 50% of patients with FI have additional behavioral or psychiatric disorders, and once those areas are addressed, FI treatment has the potential to be more successful. Tommy and his family are encouraged with this new plan of care and are hopeful for a full recovery.

Disclosure

Author has nothing to disclose.

References

[1] Colombo JM, Wassom MC, Rosen JM. Constipation and encopresis in childhood. Pediatr Rev 2015;36(9):392–401 [quiz: 402].

[2] Hyams JS, Di Lorenzo C, Saps M, et al. Functional disorders: children and adolescents. Gastroenterology 2016;150(6):1456–68.e2.

[3] Koppen IJ, von Gontard A, Chase J, et al. Management of functional nonretentive fecal incontinence in children: recommendations from the International Children's Continence Society. J Pediatr Urol 2016;12(1):56–64.

[4] Cormier D, Reilly M, Young A, et al. Encopresis plus? J Dev Behav Pediatr 2017;38(9): 772–4.

[5] DeVries M. Encopresis. In: Goldstein S, DeVries M, editors. Handbook of DSM-5 disorders in children and adolescents. Cham (Switzerland): Springer International Publishing; 2017. p. 467–80.

[6] van der Wal MF, Benninga MA, Hirasing RA. The prevalence of encopresis in a multicultural population. J Pediatr Gastroenterol Nutr 2005;40(3):345–8.

[7] Har AF, Croffie JM. Encopresis. Pediatr Rev 2010;31(9):368–74 [quiz: 374].

[8] Schonwald A, Rappaport L. Consultation with the specialist: encopresis: assessment and management. Pediatr Rev 2004;25(8):278–83.

[9] von Gontard A, Baeyens D, Van Hoecke E, et al. Psychological and psychiatric issues in urinary and fecal incontinence. J Urol 2011;185(4):1432–6.

[10] Philips EM, Peeters B, Teeuw AH, et al. Stressful life events in children with functional defecation disorders. J Pediatr Gastroenterol Nutr 2015;61(4):384–92.

[11] Davis JL. Identifying underlying emotional instability and utilizing a combined intervention in the treatment of childhood constipation and encopresis—a case report. J Altern Complement Med 2016;22(6):489–92.

[12] Lane MM, Czyzewski DI, Chumpitazi BP, et al. Reliability and validity of a modified Bristol Stool Form Scale for children. J Pediatr 2011;159(3):437–41.e1.

[13] Sood M. Functional fecal incontinence in infants and children: definition, clinical manifestations and evaluation. In: Lee S, editor. UpToDate. Waltham (MA): UptoDate; 2018 Available at: https://www.uptodate.com/contents/functional-fecal-incontinence-in-infants-and-children-definition-clinical-manifestations-and-evaluation?search=encopresis&topicRef=611&source=see_link#H10. Accessed September 4, 2019.

[14] Yang S, Chua ME, Bauer S, et al. Diagnosis and management of bladder bowel dysfunction in children with urinary tract infections: a position statement from the International Children's Continence Society. Pediatr Nephrol 2018;33(12):2207–19.

[15] Faure C, Thapar N, Di Lorenzo C. Pediatric neurogastroenterology: gastrointestinal motility and functional disorders in children. Switzerland: Springer International Publishing; 2016.

[16] Ambartsumyan L, Siddiqui A, Bauer S, et al. Simultaneous urodynamic and anorectal manometry studies in children: insights into the relationship between the lower gastrointestinal and lower urinary tracts. Neurogastroenterol Motil 2016;28(6):924–33.

[17] Sood M. Chronic functional constipation and fecal incontinence in infants and children: treatment. In: Lee S, editor. UpToDate. Waltham (MA): UptoDate; 2019. Available at: https://www.uptodate.com/contents/chronic-functional-constipation-and-fecal-incontinence-in-infants-and-children-treatment#H4. Accessed September 25, 2019.

[18] Shepard JA, Poler JE Jr, Grabman JH. Evidence-based psychosocial treatments for pediatric elimination disorders. J Clin Child Adolesc Psychol 2017;46(6):767–97.

[19] Tabbers MM, DiLorenzo C, Berger MY, et al. Evaluation and treatment of functional constipation in infants and children: evidence-based recommendations from ESPGHAN and NASPGHAN. J Pediatr Gastroenterol Nutr 2014;58(2):258–74.

[20] Wojtyniak K, Szajewska H. Systematic review: probiotics for functional constipation in children. Eur J Pediatr 2017;176(9):1155–62.

[21] Bekkali NL, van den Berg MM, Dijkgraaf MG, et al. Rectal fecal impaction treatment in childhood constipation: enemas versus high doses of oral PEG. Pediatrics 2009;124(6): e1108–15.

[22] Carter D. Conservative treatment for anal incontinence. Gastroenterol Rep (Oxf) 2014;2(2):85–91.

[23] FDA. FDA drug safety communication: FDA warns about serious heart problems with high doses of the antidiarrheal medicine loperamide (Imodium), including from abuse and misuse. FDA Drug Safety and Availability; 2018. Available at: https://www.fda.gov/drugs/drug-safety-and-availability/fda-drug-safety-communication-fda-warns-about-serious-heart-problems-high-doses-antidiarrheal. Accessed September 28, 2019.

Advances in Family Practice Nursing 2 (2020) 201–215

ADVANCES IN FAMILY PRACTICE NURSING

Screening for and Addressing Food Insecurity in the Management of Childhood Obesity

Amy Becklenberg, DNP, MSN, APRN, FNP-BC[a],*,
Tammi Tanner, EdD, MSN, CPN[a],
Wanda Csaky, DNP, APRN, FNP-BC[a],
Imelda Reyes, DNP, MPH, APRN, CPNP-PC, FNP-BC[a],
Min Jeong Jeon, MSN, RN, APRN, CPNP-PC[b],
Ashley Darcy Mahoney, PhD, APRN, NNP[b]

[a]Nell Hodgson Woodruff School of Nursing- Emory University, Office 308, 1520 Clifton Road, Atlanta, GA 30322, USA; [b]The George Washington University School of Nursing, 1919 Pennsylvania Ave. NW, Suite 500, Washington, DC 20052, USA

Keywords

• Food insecurity • Childhood obesity • Screening • Motivational interviewing
• Weight bias

Key points

• The high prevalence of food insecurity and childhood obesity negatively affects health outcomes and quality of life and often coexist.

• Advanced practice registered nurses (APRNs) and primary care clinicians are in a unique position to intervene and address both through enhanced screening and referral to appropriate resources.

• This article reviews strategies that strengthen APRN practice, including motivational interviewing and raising awareness about weight bias.

• In addition, the article provides a review of current resources, including a toolkit designed by the American Academy of Pediatrics and the Food Research & Action Center called "Addressing Food Insecurity: A Toolkit for Pediatricians."

INTRODUCTION

Childhood is an important timeframe and sets the stage for lifelong habits. Childhood obesity is a major public health problem [1] affecting approximately 18.5% of US children from the ages of 2 to 18 years [2] and has increased

*Corresponding author. E-mail address: amy.becklenberg@emory.edu

https://doi.org/10.1016/j.yfpn.2020.01.013
2589-420X/20/

dramatically since 1960. In children, overweight is defined as a body mass index (BMI) at or above the 85th percentile, and obesity is at or above the 95th percentile for children and teens of the same age and sex [3]. Almost 14% of children aged 2 to 5 years, 18.4% of children aged 6 to 11 years, and 1 in 5 adolescents are obese [2].

There are many consequences of childhood obesity including hypertension, hyperlipidemia, insulin resistance and type 2 diabetes, asthma, sleep apnea, anxiety, depression, low self-esteem, and lower self-confidence [4]. Children not only suffer biological complications but there are also social issues that affect their development. Children and adolescents with obesity have an increased risk of social problems such as bullying and stigma [4]. Furthermore, children with obesity have an increased risk of becoming an adult with obesity, which increases the risk factors for chronic diseases in adulthood [4].

Not only do children suffer from complications of obesity, but there are substantial disparities in childhood obesity among racial/ethnic minorities. Rates of obesity are higher in Black (22%) and Hispanic (25.8%) children compared with White (14.1%) children in all 3 age groups, and since 1999 the trends are increasing [2]. Asian (11%) children have the lowest prevalence [2]. There are no significant differences in prevalence of obesity by race between boys and girls [2].

In the United States, health care focuses on the treatment of disease and prevention within our current medical system. There are many ways to promote health: eating well, being physically active, receiving vaccines, avoiding smoking, and receiving preventative health check-ups. However, there are many factors that contribute to health that are not typically associated with health care. The World Health Organization defines social determinants of health as "the conditions in which people are born, grow, live, work, and age" [5]. These determinants are shaped by economic policies and systems, social norms, social policies, and political systems [5]. Social determinants of health affect a wide range of health, function, and quality-of-life outcomes and risks [6]. As a primary care provider, being able to recognize these issues during health encounters will enhance the care provided.

Population health outcomes can be significantly influenced by social health determinants. According to the United States Census Bureau, 16.2% percent of children younger than 18 years live in poverty and may have unmet needs such as a secure home environment and food security, which is exacerbated by lack of transportation and living in a food desert [7]. Another 22% live in near-poor, low-income families, and many households suffer from issues such as gaps in insurance coverage [8]. Living in poverty ultimately affects food affordability and food choices and thus the quality of food consumed [9]. Children living in poverty are significantly less likely to complete high school and complete postsecondary education than children who have never been poor [10]. A decreased educational attainment is associated with obesity. Children whose parents do not have a college degree have a significantly increased risk of being obese compared with children whose parents have a college degree [11].

Where a child lives affects the schooling experience, influence of peers, and mental health, which in turn can influence how many resources are available for families to be able to raise children. Neighborhoods with high crime rates often have increased obesity rates [12]. Conversely, neighborhoods where the streets are lined with trees are associated with a decrease in obesity [12]. Food insecurity (FI) is the "limited or uncertain access to enough food" [13]. FI is a distinctly different phenomenon than hunger. FI is typically examined at the household level, whereas hunger is an individual's sensation of pain or discomfort associated with food deprivation. Hunger may result from FI but is not necessarily the most persistent or severe result of being food insecure. One in six children live in a food insecure household [13]. Living in poverty increases the risk of FI and estimates show 2 out of 3 children living in poverty are food insecure [13]. Food assistance programs are associated with a lower risk of obesity [14]. Children living in FI households become sick more often and are hospitalized with higher frequency [13]. The relationship between obesity, which currently effects about 18.5% of our nation's children, and FI has proved complex, as families experiencing FI face many unique challenges that will be discussed later [2].

THE COEXISTENCE OF FOOD INSECURITY AND CHILDHOOD OBESITY

The coexistence of FI and childhood obesity may initially seem contradictory. Some providers may assume that if a child's BMI is high, then the child must be consistently overeating and therefore assume that food is plentiful in the home. However, in recent years, researchers have focused on gaining a deeper understanding of the causes of childhood obesity and have found that rates of childhood obesity are significantly higher in families experiencing FI.

In order to better understand the coexistence of FI and obesity, in 2010 the Institute of Medicine convened a workshop entitled "Hunger and Obesity: Understanding a Food Insecurity Paradigm," focused on the relationship between FI and obesity, given the exceedingly high rates of both in the United States [15]. Among other work done at this workshop, researchers proposed key questions and identified gaps in the knowledge base and plans for gaining a better understanding of the connection between FI and obesity [15]. One of the largest studies that highlighted the prevalence of FI and childhood obesity completed by Metallinos-Katsaras and colleagues [16] found a strong association between families experiencing FI and childhood obesity, with 28,000 low-income children within a Women, Infacts, and Children (WIC) program.

Another study that highlighted the prevalence of the coexistence of FI and childhood obesity was a recent study conducted by Oberle and colleagues [17]. In this study, all 822 participants were seeking treatment of obesity and all were screened for FI, resulting in 139 positive screens. Most of those who screened positive for FI also had severe obesity. The FI households were more likely to consume high amounts of sugar along with high-calorie, nutrient-poor foods that are often less expensive. FI also contributed to irregular eating patterns including periods of restriction and binging. When food was available, the children binged [17].

Jackson and colleagues [18] found an association between FI and obesity in a study of 186 rural elementary school–age children. FI was higher among obese children but lower if the obese child qualified for the school lunch program. Participating in the school lunch program may reduce FI by providing 1 to 2 meals a day for the children. These results establish the importance of screening all children who are overweight or obese for FI and referral to available food resources [18].

Some studies have found that the coexistence of FI and childhood obesity is more prevalent among certain ethnic groups. In a study by Papas and colleagues [19], FI was found to increase the prevalence of childhood obesity among Hispanic families. Flórez and colleagues [20] examined data from the National Health Interview Survey that included 7532 Latino youth and also found that FI was strongly associated with an increased childhood obesity prevalence.

Although children in families with FI experience some of the same risks for obesity as children in food secure families, such as large portion sizes and increased screen time [4], they experience additional risk factors as well [21]. In 2015, the Food Research & Action Center published an article entitled "Understanding the Connections: Food Insecurity and Obesity" [21]. This article summarized research findings that help explain the unique challenges faced by families experiencing FI in relation to obesity. These reasons, in addition to other previously discussed reasons, also included lack of access to grocery stores and farmer's markets where a variety of fresh fruits and vegetables are available as well as limited access to safe parks and recreational areas that provide opportunities for physical activity.

FI can affect the risk of developing obesity for children of all ages. FI increases the risk of depression among parents and caregivers, which can affect parenting practices related to infant feeding and toddler overweight [22]. In a qualitative study by Tester and colleagues [23], disordered eating behaviors among both food secure and FI children were explored. Adolescents who were in FI households endorsed hiding food and night-time snacking, which was not the case among adolescents who were in food secure households [23].

Children from families experiencing FI have been found to have a higher intake of sugar-sweetened beverages or fruit juice, as these beverages are often less expensive than milk and other healthier foods [17]. In addition, low-income communities have a higher concentration of fast food restaurants [24]. This places children at risk for increased consumption of energy-dense, nutrient-poor foods, further increasing the risk of obesity [17]. The harmful effects of FI and childhood obesity are undeniable and must be addressed by health care providers as researchers continue to explicate the reasons for this association.

SCREENING FOR FOOD INSECURITY

Because of the high prevalence of FI, in 2015 the American Academy of Pediatrics (AAP) recommended that providers screen all children for FI [25]. Screening for FI for all children normalizes this screening and minimizes the risk of families feeling "singled out," embarrassed, or ashamed that they are being asked about this sensitive topic. In addition, if health care providers only screen families they may suspect are affected by FI, they will likely miss screening families that could benefit from support due to their internal bias. Parents may try to hide FI and may have a well-dressed appearance and other possessions such as expensive cell phones and clothes [25]. Because advanced practice registered nurses (APRNs) are very effective in building trusting relationships with families, they are in an ideal position to screen families for FI and link them to resources for low-cost healthy foods.

The AAP recommends using the Hunger Vital Sign (HVS), which is a 2-question screening tool that was developed based on the 18-item Household Food Security Survey that is used by the US Department of Agriculture [26]. The HVS has a 97% sensitivity and 83% specificity and can be used by a wide range of professionals including nurse practitioners, social workers, physicians, medical assistants, and others who are trained on how to administer the HVS with sensitivity [26]. When using the HVS (2015), a positive screen is indicated if families respond "often true" or "sometimes true" to either or both statements [27]. Even if families reply "never true" to both statements, it is possible that they may still be in need of food assistance but may not yet be comfortable reporting that they are experiencing FI [27]. If families have a positive screen for FI, it is imperative that this need is addressed. In a study by Palakshappa and colleagues [28] health care providers in 6 pediatric clinics reported that time and workflow were not barriers to using the HVS screening tool and all providers viewed the screening as quick. In addition, Children's Health Watch encourages providers to use the HVS in the same way that other key vital signs are measured at each visit [29].

APRNs should begin using the HVS during prenatal visits and then with pediatric patients as early as the first newborn visit. Indeed, FI can have profound impacts on fetal origins of disease and newborn outcomes. The prevalence rates of preterm delivery in cases with mothers who experienced FI during pregnancy have been shown to be two times higher than mothers who did not experience FI during pregnancy [30]. APRNs should continue to screen families for FI at each follow-up well-child visit at 1 month, 2 months, 4 months, 6 months up to 18 years of age, as access to sufficient food can vary from month to month and can change with family changes such as job loss, family illness, and divorce [13]. The HVS screening can be done at sick visits as well, as sick visits may provide an additional opportunity for reaching families experiencing FI. Children who are experiencing FI are more likely to be sick and recover more slowly from illness and are also more likely to be hospitalized [27].

Infants and toddlers who are part of families experiencing FI are at risk for poor health outcomes. Families who cannot afford formula can often resort to the practice of watering down formula known as formula "stretching" [31]. In a study done at the Cincinnati Children's Hospital Medical Center's urban pediatric clinics (n = 144), Burkhardt and colleagues found that two-thirds of families that were enrolled in the federal Special Supplemental Nutrition WIC program ran out of WIC-supplied formula, with 27% resorting to formula stretching [31]. This can have significant health consequences on an infant's developing brain, increasing the risk for learning and behavioral and psychological problems. In a meta-analysis conducted by Moradi and colleagues [32], a positive correlation between FI and risk of anemia was found among 19 studies. One of the studies included in this meta-analysis that included 625 infants and toddlers found an association between FI and iron deficiency anemia, which can lead to poor cognitive, health, and behavioral outcomes [33]. For these reasons, it is imperative that APRNs screen for FI as early and as often as possible.

IMPLICATIONS FOR PRACTICE

There are many different strategies that healthcare professionals have used to address FI, ranging from linking families to federal assistance programs (i.e. The Special Supplemental Nutrition Program for Women, Infants, and Children (WIC), Supplemental Nutrition Assistance Program (SNAP) and the National School Lunch and National School Breakfast Programs among others) as well as local food banks and even starting food pantries on site at the health care facility [34]. In their "Addressing FI: A Toolkit for Pediatricians," the AAP and the Food Research & Action Center (FRAC) recommend a stepwise approach for health centers preparing for screening for FI (Table 1) [13]. Step 1 includes educating and training health center staff on FI and the importance of FI. They recommend identifying a "Hunger Champion" who can take the lead on identifying programs and resources, as well as increasing awareness about FI in the community. Step 2 includes implementing HVS screening at all primary care visits. If universal screening is not possible, then health care providers should be made aware of the importance of screening in special cases, such as patients who are anemic, patients whose parents mention loss of employment, patients with behavioral issues, and patients who have other medical conditions that require expensive medications [13]. Step 3 includes implementing the HVS screening tool into the electronic medical records system so that screening is easy and automatic. The HVS could be used when vital signs are taken, while the patient is waiting to see the provider, during the visit with the provider, or at any point during the visit, and can be performed by any health center staff who have been trained about screening in a sensitive manner. Step 4 in the AAP and FRAC toolkit emphasizes the importance of displaying sensitivity when screening for FI, due to the sensitive nature of the screening.

The AAP and FRAC toolkit also uses a stepwise approach to connecting patients and families to food resources (Table 2) [35]. Connecting families

Table 1
Taken verbatim from "Addressing Food Insecurity: A Toolkit for Pediatricians" developed by the American Academy of Pediatrics and the Food Research and Action Center

Preparations to screen for food insecurity	
Step 1	Educate and train leaders and staff on food insecurity and the importance of universal screening. Also, collaborate with the practice team to identify way to screen for food insecurity.
Step 2	Follow AAP's recommendation of screening at "scheduled health maintenance visits or sooner, if indicated."
Step 3	Incorporate food insecurity screening into the institutional workflow so it is sustainable, such as adding a screening tool into existing registration or intake procedures or into the electronic health record.
Step 4	Show sensitivity when screening for food insecurity (eg, inform patients that the practice screens all patients, normalize the screening tool questions).

From Addressing Food Insecurity: A Toolkit for Pediatricians. *Food Res Action Cent.* https://www.frac.org/aaptoolkit. Accessed October 29, 2019.

to local and regional food pantries can also be a valuable resource [36]. Many health centers across the United States have implemented innovative approaches to screening and addressing the needs of families experiencing FI (Table 3). However, providers need to recognize some of the barriers to using assistant programs, which may include limited English proficiency. It is important to have staff who are bilingual and bicultural to work with families who speak other languages [34].

Screening for FI during visits can help families feel comfortable about speaking about other struggles in their lives [36]. With a positive FI screen along with an overweight or obesity diagnosis, providers should assess further due to the complexity of FI problems in the family that affects both physical and mental health of the children and their families [36]. It is important to note that childhood obesity not only affects the child but also multiple family members in the household [37].

Table 2
Taken verbatim from "Addressing Food Insecurity: A Toolkit for Pediatricians" developed by the American Academy of Pediatrics and the Food Research and Action Center

Connect patients and their families to the federal nutrition programs and other food resources	
Step 1	Educate the medical team on available federal nutrition programs and emergency food resources.
Step 2	Decide who in your practice can help connect patients and their families to nutrition programs and food assistance and when you need to enlist the help of a partner.
Step 3	Post information on federal nutrition programs in your waiting room to encourage program participation.
Step 4	Assess the capacity of your practice to implement other strategies to address food insecurity.

From Addressing Food Insecurity: A Toolkit for Pediatricians. *Food Res Action Cent.* https://www.frac.org/aaptoolkit. Accessed October 29, 2019.

Table 3
Exemplar programs at health centers addressing food insecurity

Program name and city	Program description
Chicago: The Rush Surplus Project at Rush University Medical Center	Repackages hospital food that would otherwise be discarded and donates this food to local shelters in the community as well as local high school and a YMCA.
Minnesota: Hennepin County Medical Center (HCMC) and Second Harvest Hartland partnership	A pediatrician developed a relationship between the health center and one of the largest food banks in the United States. HCMC screens patients for FI using the HVS. They implemented a referral system that connects patients who screen positive for FI with nutrition resources in the community. Citation: CHW_HVS_whitepaper_FINAL.pdf. https://childrenshealthwatch.org/wp-content/uploads/CHW_HVS_whitepaper_FINAL.pdf. Accessed October 7, 2019.
Boston: Grow Clinic at Boston Medical Center	First hospital in the United States to open a food pantry on-site; began with one pediatrician who had a food pantry in her desk drawer. They now train pediatric medical residents on how to ask about FI using "normative phrasing" to increase skill in how to assess appropriately and compassionately.
Atlanta: CHOA Strong4Life clinic	Assess every family at the initial visit and again at the 4th visit for FI using the HVS tool. If family screens positive, they are given a flyer for United Way of Greater Atlanta 2-1-1. The family can call this number any time, any day and be confidentially connected to resources for basic needs, education, income, health, and homelessness.

Data from Citation: Grenier J, Wynn N. A Nurse-Led Intervention to Address Food Insecurity in Chicago.-Online J Issues Nurs. 2018;23(3):1-1. https://doi.org/10.3912/OJIN.Vol23No03Man04) and CHW_HVS_whitepaper_FINAL.pdf.https://childrenshealthwatch.org/wp-content/uploads/CHW_HVS_whitepaper_FINAL.pdf. Accessed October 7, 2019.

WEIGHT BIAS

Weight bias includes attitudes, judgments, and assumptions based on negative stereotypes of people with obesity. Depression and anxiety, especially from worrying about bullying, are associated with weight bias. Because of the experiences people with obesity go through, they often have lower quality of life and a negative impact on their overall well-being [8].

Many believe using shame and blame will motivate an overweight child or adolescent to lose weight. This stigma actually leads to more disordered eating such as binge eating, social isolation, and decreased physical activity. It also has a significant impact on the quality of life [38]. Many studies have suggested that health care professionals, even those working with obesity, exhibit weight bias. Perpetuating stereotypes of patients with obesity, assuming they have no self-control, and that they are lazy, can lead to a decrease in health-seeking behaviors [39].

In 2017, The AAP issued a policy statement about weight stigma to raise awareness of the prevalence and negative effects. The recommendations include modeling best practices for nonbiased language and behaviors in the clinic; using empathetic counseling techniques such as motivational interviewing; addressing any issues the patient/family may have with weight bias or bullying at each visit; being an advocate for weight stigma education for health professionals; and empowering families to address weight bias in their home and communities [40].

Individuals with obesity often experience similar bias and discrimination as marginalized racial or ethnic groups and the lesbian, gay, bisexual, and transgender communities [41]. This can result in a decrease in health-seeking behaviors. Weight bias can also have psychological effects on individuals. It can lead to disordered eating, lack of interest in physical activity, and increased caloric intake [42]. Not eating in front of other people, not traveling because the seatbelt on the plane will not fit, and not going to the beach because they do not want others to see them in a swimsuit are some examples of how people with obesity avoid social situations [43].

It is important for medical providers to understand the impact of their weight bias. Language and actual physical barriers can stigmatize patients and have a negative effect. Ensuring patients "fit" physically in the clinic setting is very important. Larger examination tables, chairs, and appropriate scales to weigh in private places not only make the visit more comfortable but also let the patient know you can care for them safely [44]. Providing a safe, nonjudgmental environment where patients with obesity can seek medical care can lead to positive health outcomes [45].

The language used by health care providers can increase the stigma associated with obesity. A sample of 1064 residents of the United States rated 10 terms to determine if the words were desirable, stigmatizing, blaming, or motivating. *Weight* and *unhealthy weight* were reported as the participants' most desirable terms for health care providers to use. *Fat* and *morbidly obese* were rated as the most undesirable terms to use when discussing weight-related issues [39]. These results were consistent across socioeconomic classes. It was also reported that 19% stated they would not seek medical attention after having a stigmatizing experience.

Health care providers have a responsibility to interact with patients in a respectful, nonblaming way. Being aware of how language can affect patients is an important factor when caring for people with obesity [39]. The Yale Rudd Center for Food Policy and Obesity offer many resources to help increase awareness of weight bias in health care professionals. Raising awareness of personal biases would help to decrease the chance of those biases affecting clinical care. A brief video, *Weight Bias in Healthcare*, was used to study weight bias in second- and third-year medical students [46]. Three measures were used to measure weight bias before and after viewing the video. The measures included Fat Phobia Scale, the Attitudes toward Obese Persons Scale, and the Beliefs about Obese Persons Scale. The results showed viewing the brief video had a decrease in the negative stereotypes related to people with obesity. Lee and colleagues [47] recommended many types of interventions to decrease weight bias. Learning about the multiple causes, role playing exercises, videos, and using standardized patients can show a decrease in the negative stereotyping of this population [47,48].

The AAP published an algorithm for the assessment and management of childhood obesity in patients aged 2 years and older [49]. Depending on the patients' weight classification, providers should determine the next treatment plan [49]. Multidisciplinary programs such as Strong4Life by Children's Healthcare of Atlanta provides counseling to individuals through motivational interviewing to screen for barriers and nutritional assessment to help teach families on choosing nutritious foods and set physical activity goals when lower levels of physical activity are reported with FI [37]. Follow-up visits with a nutritionist to address FI among obese pediatric patients can help empower families to make healthy food choices. In addition, referral to healthy food resources can decrease family stress due to uncertain availability of food [30]. Referral to a mental health provider will help address not only pediatric patient's emotional stress related to obesity but also family members' stress with FI. It is essential for providers to screen and provide guidance for pediatric patients and their families experiencing FI, as risk of FI increases with parental anxiety, substance abuse, moderate-to-severe maternal depression, and households with complex structures such as a cohabitating adult [36]. Moreover, FI can lead to poor school performance and increased behavioral and emotional problems for children aged 4 to 18 years [50]. In addition, school-age children experiencing FI are at risk for poor school performance, especially in math and reading, as well as aggression, depression, and anxiety [51,52].

MOTIVATIONAL INTERVIEWING

Primary care providers have expressed they lack strategies to discuss health concerns with overweight and obese patients [53]. Motivational interviewing (MI) is a patient-centered approach to counseling families with obesity. This technique uses support, open-ended questions, reflective listening and shared decision-making and also helps to prompt change talk [54]. MI uses several empathetic strategies to develop a collaborative strategy to elicit change. The acronym OARS is used for these strategies:

- O: open ended questions,
- A: affirmations,
- R: reflective listening, and
- S: summary statements.

By working with the patient/family, the provider demonstrates respect and a partnership leading to a more therapeutic relationship [55].

A randomized study done in 42 practices compared 3 groups. The first used their usual methods to care for overweight and obese children. The second group saw only the provider and had 4 MI counseling sessions. Group 3 saw the provider and the registered dietitian (RD) and had 4 MI sessions with the provider and 6 MI sessions with the RD. The children were observed over 2 years. After 2 years, the group 3 participants had significantly lower BMI percentiles [56].

The use of motivational interviewing has been linked to lower rates of provider burnout and improved patient satisfaction in clinics [57]. Some providers have expressed the concern that MI will be more time consuming and not worth the effort. It has been shown to be an effective tool to use, with patients trying to make lifestyle changes. With proper training and practice, the health care teams will become proficient in this technique [58]. In one study, MI was taught to staff and clinicians to study the impact on clinician communication and patient satisfaction. The results showed that coaching in MI techniques resulted in a reduction in clinician burnout, a decrease in barriers for discussing behavior changes, and clinicians improved their self-rated MI skills [57].

New MI providers would benefit from practicing with role-playing or audio-taped interviews. It is also recommended that before each interview, the provider take a moment to think about the specific strategies they would like to use. Formal training in motivational interviewing for the entire clinic team can also be valuable [59].

MI builds on intrinsic motivation. A study done with children in an after-school program and health coaches used MI to help the children work through barriers and set goals to improve their eating and exercise. The health coaches had 9 goal setting sessions with the elementary school children. They met weekly, set goals for the next week, reviewed progress on last week's goals, and participated in a group exercise activity and healthy eating activity. The children all reported improved eating and exercise habits [60].

MI gives the medical provider the opportunity to work with patients as a team. If adolescents come to the provider with feelings of ambivalence and the provider can work with them instead of confronting, it can lead to improved outcomes. Treating the adolescent with respect and working with them as a partner, the adolescent will feel more autonomy. This may increase adherence to the program, which would also lead to improved health this population. Bean, and colleagues [61] studied adolescents enrolled in T.E.EN.S., a weight management program. The participants were randomized to MI or control. The control continued with the usual treatment—biweekly dietitian and behavioral support visits—along with 3 times a week supervised physical activity. The teens in the MI group demonstrated greater treatment adherence than the control group. There was a high attrition rate (20.6%) before the first MI session. These investigators recommend using MI before the start of treatment to assess readiness and motivation to change behaviors [61].

When presenting target behaviors to the patient and family, the provider should stress the importance that the recommendations are for the entire family, not just the one child who is overweight. Using MI to help the family determine what behaviors they are ready to change and then to make small goals to achieve that change is empowering to families [62].

SUMMARY

APRNs will inevitably encounter a high prevalence of patients experiencing both childhood obesity and FI. APRNs and nurses seeing patients in a multitude of health care settings are uniquely situated to identify and address the complex social problem of FI, especially when working with patients experiencing childhood obesity [63]. Indeed, family nurse practitioners, pediatric nurse practitioners, and registered nurses are in an ideal position to screen children and families for FI and then link patients to myriad resources [63]. Successful nurse-led FI interventions have shown success both at the individual patient level and at a system level [63,64].

It is imperative that APRNs increase their knowledge and skills for more effectively addressing the factors contributing to both of these interrelated conditions. In particular, routinely screening patients and families for FI is an important start. A 2012 survey of health care providers (medical doctors and nurse practitioners) by Hoisington and colleagues [65] found that fewer than 25% of respondents routinely inquired about household food quality and fewer than 13% routinely inquired about household food sufficiency; however, 88% of clinicians said they would be willing to do so. This willingness must translate into universal screening of all pediatric patients and families in an effort to optimize their growth and development. It is especially imperative that families with pediatric patients with high BMI receive screening for FI and extra sensitivity regarding the unique challenges they may face. Handouts and links to resources include contact information for public programs or other low-cost interventions that APRNs can use in their practice settings. Working together providers can leverage their unique and complementary skills, expertise, and resources to synergistically address FI and childhood obesity.

Disclosure

None of the above authors have any commercial or financial conflicts of interest. There are no funding sources for this article.

References
[1] Childhood obesity facts | Overweight &obesity | CDC. 2019. Available at: https://www.cdc.gov/obesity/data/childhood.html. Accessed October 17, 2019.

[2] Hales C. Data briefs prevalence of obesity among adults and youth: United States, 2015–2016 - number 288 - October 2017. 2019. Available at: https://www.cdc.gov/nchs/products/databriefs/db288.htm. Accessed October 17, 2019.

[3] Defining childhood obesity | Overweight &obesity | CDC. 2019. Available at: https://www.cdc.gov/obesity/childhood/defining.html. Accessed October 17, 2019.

[4] CDC. Causes and consequences of childhood obesity. Centers for Disease Control and Prevention; 2016. Available at: https://www.cdc.gov/obesity/childhood/causes.html. Accessed October 17, 2019.

[5] WHO | Commission on Social Determinants of Health - final report. WHO. Available at: http://www.who.int/social_determinants/thecommission/finalreport/en/. Accessed October 17, 2019.

[6] Social Determinants of Health | Healthy People 2020. Available at: https://www.healthy-people.gov/2020/topics-objectives/topic/social-determinants-of-health/objectives. Accessed October 17, 2019.

[7] Garg A, Cull W, Olson L, et al. Screening and referral for low-income families' social determinants of health by US pediatricians. Acad Pediatr 2019; https://doi.org/10.1016/j.acap.2019.05.125.

[8] Beck AF, Henize AW, Kahn RS, et al. Forging a pediatric primary care-community partnership to support food-insecure families. Pediatrics 2014;134(2):e564–571.

[9] Sturm R, Datar A. Regional price differences and food consumption frequency among elementary school children. Public Health 2011;125(3):136–41.

[10] Ratcliffe C. Child poverty and adult success. Urban Institute; 2016. Available at: https://www.urban.org/research/publication/child-poverty-and-adult-success. Accessed October 17, 2019.

[11] Singh GK, Siahpush M, Kogan MD. Rising social inequalities in US childhood obesity, 2003-2007. Ann Epidemiol 2010;20(1):40–52.

[12] Lovasi GS, Schwartz-Soicher O, Quinn JW, et al. Neighborhood safety and green space as predictors of obesity among preschool children from low-income families in New York City. Prev Med 2013;57(3):189–93.

[13] Addressing food insecurity: a toolkit for pediatricians. Food Res Action Cent. Available at: https://www.frac.org/aaptoolkit. Accessed October 29, 2019.

[14] Carrillo-Larco RM, Miranda JJ, Bernabé-Ortiz A. Impact of food assistance programs on obesity in mothers and children: a prospective cohort study in Peru. Am J Public Health 2016;106(7):1301–7.

[15] Hou S-I. Hunger and obesity: understanding a food insecurity paradigm. Health Promot Pract 2013;14(3):317–20.

[16] Metallinos-Katsaras E, Must A, Gorman K. A longitudinal study of food insecurity on obesity in preschool children. J Acad Nutr Diet 2012;112(12):1949–58.

[17] Oberle MM, Romero Willson S, Gross AC, et al. Relationships among child eating behaviors and household food insecurity in youth with obesity. Child Obes 2019;15(5):298–305.

[18] Jackson JA, Smit E, Branscum A, et al. The family home environment, food insecurity, and body mass index in rural children. Health Educ Behav 2017;44(4):648–57.

[19] Papas MA, Trabulsi JC, Dahl A, et al. Food insecurity increases the odds of obesity among young hispanic children. J Immigr Minor Health 2016;18(5):1046–52.

[20] Flórez KR, Katic BJ, López-Cevallos DF, et al. The double burden of food insecurity and obesity among Latino youth: understanding the role of generational status. Pediatr Obes 2019;14(9):e12525.

[21] Understanding the connections: food insecurity and obesity (October 2015). Food Res Action Cent. Available at: https://frac.org/research/resource-library/understanding-connections-food-insecurity-obesity. Accessed November 27, 2019.

[22] Bronte-Tinkew J, Zaslow M, Capps R, et al. Food insecurity works through depression, parenting, and infant feeding to influence overweight and health in toddlers. J Nutr 2007;137(9):2160–5.

[23] Tester JM, Lang TC, Laraia BA. Disordered eating behaviours and food insecurity: a qualitative study about children with obesity in low-income households. Obes Res Clin Pract 2016;10(5):544–52.

[24] Fleischhacker SE, Evenson KR, Rodriguez DA, et al. A systematic review of fast food access studies. Obes Rev 2011;12(5):e460–71.

[25] AAP Department of Community. New toolkit helps pediatricians address food insecurity in patients. AAP News 2019. https://www.aappublications.org/news/2017/05/31/Chapters053117. Accessed September 17, 2019.

[26] Hager ER, Quigg AM, Black MM, et al. Development and validity of a 2-item screen to identify families at risk for food insecurity. Pediatrics 2010;126(1):e26–32.

[27] O'Keefe L. Identifying food insecurity: two-question screening tool has 97% sensitivity. AAP News 2015; https://doi.org/10.1542/aapnews.20151023-1.

[28] Palakshappa D, Doupnik S, Vasan A, et al. Suburban families' experience with food insecurity screening in primary care practices. Pediatrics 2017;140(1); https://doi.org/10.1542/peds.2017-0320.

[29] CHW_HVS_whitepaper_FINAL.pdf. Available at: https://childrenshealthwatch.org/wp-content/uploads/CHW_HVS_whitepaper_FINAL.pdf. Accessed October 7, 2019.

[30] Dolatian M, Sharifi N, Mahmoodi Z. Relationship of socioeconomic status, psychosocial factors, and food insecurity with preterm labor: a longitudinal study. Int J Reprod Biomed 2018;16(9):563–70.

[31] Burkhardt MC, Beck AF, Kahn RS, et al. Are our babies hungry? Food insecurity among infants in urban clinics. Clin Pediatr (Phila) 2012;51(3):238–43.

[32] Moradi S, Arghavani H, Issah A, et al. Food insecurity and anaemia risk: a systematic review and meta-analysis. Public Health Nutr 2018;21(16):3067–79.

[33] Skalicky A, Meyers AF, Adams WG, et al. Child food insecurity and iron deficiency anemia in low-income infants and toddlers in the United States. Matern Child Health J 2006;10(2): 177–85.

[34] Council on Community Pediatrics, Committee on Nutrition. Promoting food security for all children. Pediatrics 2015;136(5):e1431–8.

[35] Gilbert D, Nanda J, Paige D. Securing the safety net: concurrent participation in income eligible assistance programs. Matern Child Health J 2014;18(3):604–12.

[36] Walsh SM, Palmer W, Welsh JA, et al. Challenges and successes of a multidisciplinary pediatric obesity treatment program. NutrClinPract 2014;29(6):780–5.

[37] Browne NT. Food insecurity: assessment and intervention. J Pediatr Surg Nurs 2017;6(1): 7–10.

[38] Callahan D. Children, stigma, and obesity. JAMA Pediatr 2013;167(9):791–2.

[39] Puhl R, Peterson JL, Luedicke J. Fighting obesity or obese persons? Public perceptions of obesity-related health messages. Int J Obes 2013;37(6):774–82.

[40] Pont SJ, Puhl R, Cook SR, et al. stigma experienced by children and adolescents with obesity. Pediatrics 2017;140(6):e20173034.

[41] Halvorson EE, Curley T, Wright M, et al. Weight bias in pediatric inpatient care. Acad Pediatr 2019;19(7):780–6.

[42] Schvey NA, White MA. The internalization of weight bias is associated with severe eating pathology among lean individuals. Eat Behav 2015;17:1–5.

[43] Carmona J, Tornero-Quiñones I, Sierra-Robles Á. Body image avoidance behaviors in adolescence: A multilevel analysis of contextual effects associated with the physical education class. Psychol Sport Exerc 2015;16:70–8.

[44] Phelan SM, Burgess DJ, Yeazel MW, et al. Impact of weight bias and stigma on quality of care and outcomes for patients with obesity. Obes Rev 2015;16(4):319–26.

[45] Sylvetsky AC, Welsh JA, Walsh SM, et al. Action-oriented obesity counseling attains weight stabilization and improves liver enzymes among overweight and obese children and adolescents. Open J Pediatr 2012;02(03):236–43.

[46] Poustchi Y, Saks NS, Piasecki AK, et al. Brief intervention effective in reducing weight bias in medical students. Fam Med 2013;45(5):345–8.

[47] Lee M, Ata RN, Brannick MT. Malleability of weight-biased attitudes and beliefs: a meta-analysis of weight bias reduction interventions. Body Image 2014;11(3):251–9.

[48] Kushner RF, Zeiss DM, Feinglass JM, et al. An obesity educational intervention for medical students addressing weight bias and communication skills using standardized patients. BMC Med Educ 2014;14(1):53.

[49] Eisenmann JC, Gundersen C, Lohman BJ, et al. Is food insecurity related to overweight and obesity in children and adolescents? A summary of studies, 1995-2009: Food insecurity and obesity in children. Obes Rev 2011;12(5):e73–83.

[50] New AAP report targets lack of adequate food as ongoing health risk to U.S. children. Available at: https://www.aap.org/en-us/about-the-aap/aap-press-room/Pages/Lack-of-Adequate-Food.aspx. Accessed October 30, 2019.

[51] Gundersen C, Ziliak JP. Childhood food insecurity in the U.S.: trends, causes, and policy options. Future Child 2014;24(2):1–19.

[52] Jyoti DF, Frongillo EA, Jones SJ. Food insecurity affects school children's academic performance, weight gain, and social skills. J Nutr 2005;135(12):2831–9.

[53] Steeves JA, Liu B, Willis G, et al. Physicians' personal beliefs about weight-related care and their associations with care delivery: The U.S. National Survey of Energy Balance Related Care among Primary Care Physicians. Obes Res Clin Pract 2015;9(3):243–55.

[54] Anderson KL. A review of the prevention and medical management of childhood obesity. Child Adolesc Psychiatr Clin 2018;27(1):63–76.

[55] Kennedy D, Apodaca T, Trowbridge K, et al. Learning motivational interviewing: a pathway to caring and mindful patient encounters. J Pediatr Nurs 2016;31(5):505–10.

[56] Resnicow K, Sonneville KR, Naar S. The heterogeneity of MI interventions studies for treatment of obesity. Pediatrics 2018;142(5):e20182471.

[57] Pollak KI, Nagy P, Bigger J, et al. Effect of teaching motivational interviewing via communication coaching on clinician and patient satisfaction in primary care and pediatric obesity-focused offices. Patient Educ Couns 2016;99(2):300–3.

[58] Brobeck E, Bergh H, Odencrants S, et al. Primary healthcare nurses' experiences with motivational interviewing in health promotion practice. J Clin Nurs 2011;20(23–24):3322–30.

[59] Borrello M, Pietrabissa G, Ceccarini M, et al. Motivational interviewing in childhood obesity treatment. Front Psychol 2015;6; https://doi.org/10.3389/fpsyg.2015.01732.

[60] Ige TJ, DeLeon P, Nabors L. Motivational Interviewing in an obesity prevention program for children. Health Promot Pract 2017;18(2):263–74.

[61] Bean MK, Ingersoll KS, Powell P, et al. Impact of motivational interviewing on outcomes of an adolescent obesity treatment: results from the MI Values randomized controlled pilot trial. Clin Obes 2018;8(5):323–6.

[62] Brown CL, Perrin EM. Obesity prevention and treatment in primary care. Acad Pediatr 2018;18(7):736–45.

[63] Kersten HB, Beck AF, Klein M, editors. Identifying and addressing childhood food insecurity in healthcare and community settings. Cham (Switzerland): Springer International Publishing; 2018; https://doi.org/10.1007/978-3-319-76048-3.

[64] Grenier J, Wynn N. A nurse-led intervention to address food insecurity in Chicago. Online J Issues Nurs 2018;23(3):1.

[65] Hoisington AT, Braverman MT, Hargunani DE, et al. Health care providers' attention to food insecurity in households with children. Prev Med 2012;55(3):219–22.

Advances in Family Practice Nursing 2 (2020) 217–225

ADVANCES IN FAMILY PRACTICE NURSING

ELSEVIER
MOSBY

Addressing Human Papillomavirus Prevention and Vaccine Hesitancy

Meara Henley, DNP, MSN, RN, CPNP, PMHS

North County Health Services, 150 Valpreda Road, San Marcos, CA 92069, USA

Keywords

- HPV vaccine • HPV vaccine hesitancy • Increasing HPV vaccination rates
- HPV prevention • High-quality HPV vaccine recommendation
- Building trust with parents regarding HPV vaccination

Key points

- Despite the importance of preventing human papillomavirus (HPV) via vaccination, overall adolescent vaccination rates remain low, potentially due to HPV vaccine–hesitant parents.
- HPV vaccine hesitancy can be counteracted by providing high-quality recommendations from providers regarding parental concerns.
- Commonly cited HPV vaccine concerns include vaccine safety, efficacy, and potential for increase in sexual activity.
- HPV vaccine hesitancy also can be addressed by starting early, presenting HPV vaccine with authority, being honest about side effects, building trust, and focusing on prevention.

INTRODUCTION

Human papillomavirus (HPV) is a well-established source of most cervical and anogenital cancers. HPV is found in specific tissue types that include carcinomas of the cervix and squamous cell cancers (SCCs) of the vulva, vagina, penis, oropharynx, and anus [1]. After much research and testing, in 2006 a quadrivalent vaccine was approved by the Food and Drug Administration to address HPV infections, and provide protection against HPV-associated cancers and HPV-related warts [2]. This was followed by the approval of the 9-valent HPV vaccine in 2014 [2,3]. In the United States, the Centers for Disease

E-mail address: meara.henley@nchs-health.org

https://doi.org/10.1016/j.yfpn.2020.01.008

Control and Prevention (CDC) began recommending administration of the HPV vaccine for girls in 2006, and expanded this recommendation to boys in 2011 [2,4]. The administration of the HPV vaccine has decreased the number of HPV-associated cancers reported yearly since its inception [5]. During 2001 to 2014, cervical carcinoma rates decreased among women aged 15 to 34 years. On average, the data showed that a 29% decrease in cervical cancer rates was noted in girls and women aged 15 to 24 years and a 13% decrease for women aged 25 to 34 years. Cervical carcinoma rates and vaginal SCCs decreased as well, with a notable sharp decline after 2009 [6]. In addition, high-risk sexual behaviors were noted to have not declined, leading to the conclusion that the dropping infection rates were in part due to the HPV vaccine [5,6].

Although the rates of HPV-associated cancers have decreased, the overall adolescent vaccination rate has remained disappointingly low. In 2016, only 43.4% of adolescents were up to date with their HPV vaccines, which was only half of the target Healthy People 2020 goal of 80% [7]. Data collected again in 2018 revealed the HPV vaccination rate at 51% overall, which was an increase of 2% since 2017 [8]. CDC data from 2017 indicated 66% of adolescents ages 13 to 17 had received the first dose of the vaccine series. The percentage of teens who started the HPV series increased on average 5% each year over the past 5 years. Although there has been an increase in the overall vaccination percentages, approximately half of adolescents have not completed the series. In addition, vaccination rates are higher in urban areas versus rural areas by approximately 7% [9]. There are many reasons for decreased HPV vaccination rates, some of which are related to vaccination hesitancy in general, and some specific to the HPV vaccination itself [10]. This article attempts to address HPV vaccine hesitancy and strategies to help improve HPV vaccination rates.

VACCINATION HESITANCY IN GENERAL

Parental concern regarding vaccinations can at worst lead to refusal of the vaccine, or at best, vaccine delay or alternative scheduling of vaccines [11,12]. Although there are many reasons for vaccine hesitancy, commonly cited apprehensions include information issues, vaccine effectiveness, immune system concerns, belief there are too many vaccines, issues of trust, and fear of injections [13]. Interestingly, parents who refuse vaccinations tend to be more educated in general, whereas those who accept vaccinations without protest or requests for more information tend to have a lower educational level. This is likely due to parental belief and supposition they are knowledgeable regarding vaccination due to personal research via the Internet or friends and family in comparison to those parents who trust their provider's recommendation without independent scrutiny. Studies also show that vaccine hesitancy often includes multiple intertwined factors and it is unlikely that a single intervention will fully address the issue [14]. Although reasons behind vaccination hesitancy are multifactorial, studies regarding vaccine hesitancy indicate that provider recommendations can greatly influence the decisions these parents make regarding vaccinations in lieu of specific disease or vaccine knowledge [12]. Parents who feel overwhelmed or uninformed regarding vaccinations may perceive vaccinations as new, ineffective, or potentially harmful [15]. For this reason, providing a strong and concrete recommendation is essential for success in vaccination rates, particularly when there is the potential for mistrust or misinformation, as is common with the HPV vaccine.

PARENTAL CONCERN WITH HUMAN PAPILLOMAVIRUS VACCINATION SPECIFICALLY

Many of the reasons for HPV vaccine hesitancy are identical to the reasoning for hesitancy of other vaccinations; however, a few reasons are specific to the HPV vaccine. As the HPV vaccine has been in the news frequently and often featured in social media, many parents are more aware of the perceived risks of the HPV vaccination as it specifically relates to certain concerns regarding the vaccine; that is, vaccine safety, length of time on the market, and issues related to sexual behavior [16]. More than half of parents reported refusal and delay because of belief that their child was not sexually active and/or does not need the vaccine at this time because they were far from sexual activity [17]. Many parents believe that protecting against HPV via vaccination will provide a green light or permission for sexual activity, or encourage unprotected sexual activity due to decreased concern for HPV transmission, although there are many studies that describe the contrary [18]. For many parents, the HPV vaccine is a new and novel vaccine, which they report does not inspire confidence. Parents additionally may feel that it is a marketing tool by pharmaceutical companies and is not necessary [19].

With vaccinations, it is important to note the difference between refusal and hesitancy. Parents may be hesitant regarding the vaccine in the 11-year to 12-year age group, but amenable when their adolescent is older. These parents are ideal for a targeted information campaign to help them realize the benefit of vaccinating in this younger age group, namely, to ensure a robust immune response before exposure to the HPV virus. Studies have shown that parents of female adolescents are more likely to express concern regarding the safety and side effects of the HPV vaccine in comparison with parents of male adolescents [20]. Armed with this knowledge, providers can anticipate these questions and come prepared to discuss and address parents' concerns. Providing high-quality recommendations specifically regarding the HPV vaccine has been shown to increase same-day vaccination rates [21]. A 2015 workgroup examined what constitutes a high-quality recommendation. The group concluded that a high-quality recommendation should contain 4 parts: timeliness (routinely recommending the vaccine at CDC-recommended ages), consistency (recommending for all eligible adolescents), urgency (the importance of vaccinating today without delay), and strength (using language that clearly conveyed that the provider believes the vaccine to be very important) [22].

In addition, there are other strategies to help increase HPV vaccine administration rates that are reported in the literature both anecdotally and through scientific study. Studies indicate that there are common questions parents have regarding the HPV vaccination (Table 1). Many of these questions have roots in concerns regarding the HPV vaccine safety and efficacy. Answering these questions can sometimes be difficult for providers who feel unprepared or less knowledgeable about the HPV vaccine [23].

Table 1
Suggested talking points for discussing human papillomavirus (HPV) with parents

"Why does my child need the HPV vaccine?"	The HPV vaccine is important because it prevents against infections that can cause cancer.
"How do you know the vaccine works?"	Studies continue to prove that the HPV vaccination works and has decreased the number of infections and HPV precancers in young people since its introduction in 2004
"Why do you recommend the vaccine at such a young age?"	Vaccines are given to protect your child before they are exposed. We give the HPV vaccine at ages 11–12 to provide protection to kids long before they are exposed. Also, if your child has the shot now, he or she will need only 2 doses. If we wait, the child may need 3.
"Do boys need the vaccine?"	The HPV vaccine protects against penile, anal, and head and neck cancers. It's just as important for boys to receive the vaccine as it is for girls.
"What diseases are caused by HPV?"	HPV can cause cancer, such as cervical, penile, anal, and head and neck cancers. But HPV can also cause genital warts.
"Is my child really at risk for HPV?"	HPV is a very common infection in women and men that can cause cancer. Almost 79 million Americans have an HPV infection with 14 million new cases each year.
"I'm worried this will make my child think it's ok to have sex"	Studies show that getting the HPV vaccine doesn't make it more likely that kids will start having sex. I made sure to vaccinate my child/grandchild and recommend the vaccine for my friends and family.
"Is this vaccine safe?"	Yes, the HPV vaccine is very safe. Like any medication, vaccines can cause side effects such as pain, swelling, or redness where the shot was given. That's normal for the HPV vaccine and other vaccines and should go away in a day or two. Rarely, kids can faint after getting the HPV vaccine, so we'll have your child stay seated or lie down for a bit after getting the vaccine to protect them.
"Can the HPV vaccine cause infertility?"	This is a common question! No evidence exists that shows that the HPV vaccine causes infertility. In fact, it prevents against HPV-associated cancers that could limit the ability to have children due to necessary treatments.

Adapted from Centers for Disease Control. Human Papillomavirus. Answering Parent Questions. Talking to Parents about the HPV Vaccine. Available at: https://www.cdc.gov/hpv/hcp/answering-questions.html.

ADDRESSING HUMAN PAPILLOMAVIRUS VACCINE HESITANCY

Start early

Discussing HPV vaccination during well-child visits is appropriate beginning a few years before the vaccine is due to be administered. Providing the CDC vaccination schedule infographic or another easy-to-read graph or chart that shows HPV vaccine recommendations helps prepare parents and families and normalize HPV vaccination [24]. Remind parents that administering the HPV vaccine at the recommended age range of 11 to 12 years will ensure a robust immune response and long-lasting protection against the HPV virus [21].

Present human papillomavirus vaccines with the same authority as other vaccines

The CDC and numerous studies recommend a presumptive approach with regard to immunization discussions, and research supports the idea that parents are more likely to accept vaccine recommendations when presented in a presumptive format. When providers restate original recommendations after addressing concerns, parents were more likely to accept recommendations [22]. Rather than querying parents about whether or not they would like the HPV vaccination, instead include the HPV vaccine with other routine immunizations for their child's age group. In addition, parents are more likely to interpret the first vaccine discussed as the most important; therefore, by listing the HPV vaccination first in the description of vaccines for which a child is due, parents may be more amenable to HPV vaccination [24].

Be honest about side effects, reassure about robust immune system

Vaccine serious events are extremely rare [3]. Parents often have concerns regarding severe side effects that have been discussed on social media or in their friend groups [25]. Perceived risk may be mitigated by discussing potential minor side effects such as muscle soreness, arm redness, or mild elevation in temperature, and reviewing that serious adverse events are extremely rare, and equal to those of other childhood immunizations [26]. Depending on the parent or family, providing information from the Vaccine Adverse Event Reporting System (VAERS) regarding HPV vaccinations may be helpful. As of 2018, a characterization of the VAERS database for HPV vaccinations from 2009 to 2015 showed that VAERS received 19,760 reports after HPV vaccination, of which 94.2% of reports were nonserious, such as dizziness, syncope, or injection site reactions. Headache, fatigue, and nausea were commonly reported in the serious adverse event category. More than 60 million HPV doses were distributed during the 2009 to 2015 period that was reviewed, and among 29 verified reports of death, there was no pattern of clustering of deaths by diagnosis, comorbidities, age, or interval from vaccination to death [27]. These data lead the authors to conclude that no new or unexpected safety concerns or reporting patterns with clinically important adverse events were detected and that the safety profile of the HPV vaccine was consistent with data from prelicensure trials and postmarketing safety data [28,29].

Build trust with parents

Studies indicate that parental trust is strengthened when a provider spends time discussing vaccines in a nonjudgmental and nonderisive manner and provides an empathetic response to concerns and questions [14,18,25]. Attempting to understand why the parent and family feel hesitant regarding vaccinations can provide information to the provider regarding the most effective approach to countering vaccine misinformation and apprehension [18]. To build trust, providers should remember that parents and teens are seeking credible information to make decisions about their health; they just want to be heard and respected [30].

Tell stories to help make vaccinations approachable

Personal stories of vaccination have demonstrated efficacy in convincing vaccine-hesitant parents by providing anecdotal evidence that providers believe in vaccines and recommend them for their friends and family [24]. In an age of social media, where a story with no scientific basis or fact can go viral in minutes, and where antivaccine advocates have a large social media presence and followers, sharing personal stories provides an opportunity to counter false information with personal statements regarding vaccine safety and vaccination belief [19]. Ideally, telling stories to make vaccination more approachable will build trust between provider and parents [31].

Focus on human papillomavirus prevention and protection

Anecdotally, parents are often interested in HPV vaccine protection in the framework of "future proofing"; that is, we cannot predict what a future partner will bring to a relationship. Parents often declare that their child will not be exposed; however, discussing future relationships tends to provide more support and reasoning for the vaccine. In addition, it provides a platform for the discussion of herd immunity and protecting those that cannot have the vaccine due to immune deficiencies, for example [17,32]. Upward of 79 million Americans are currently infected with HPV and approximately 14 million people become newly infected each year, meaning that almost every person who is sexually active will be exposed and potentially contract HPV at some point in their life if they are unvaccinated. Because HPV is spread through sexual contact, the potential for transmission exists during any sexual activity. HPV can be transmitted when asymptomatic, which is potentially problematic. The HPV vaccination is the most effective way to prevent HPV infection, followed by safe sex practices, such as condom usage and mutual monogamy [33,34].

A strategy that probably does not work

Because vaccination has been so successful, many parents are not familiar with or have not experienced particular diseases [29,33]. An idea to help counter this involves providing graphic descriptions or pictures of potential side effects or sequelae of vaccine-preventable diseases, particularly HPV. Many printed clinic materials exist with rather graphic photos of genital warts and other HPV-associated lesions. Interestingly, several studies indicate that fear appeals or scare tactics can have a negative effect on parental attitudes regarding the vaccine. Although it appears counterintuitive, framing HPV vaccination appeals with fearmongering is unlikely to sway vaccine-hesitant parents toward agreeing to vaccinate [35–39].

SUMMARY

Vaccine hesitancy, especially HPV vaccine hesitancy, is a common and important issue both for individual and community health [7]. With so many people infected with HPV, and such potential existing for infection, vaccination is crucial to personal and public health. This is in direct contradiction to the current adolescent vaccination rates [8,9]. Facts alone are often not sufficient to change the opinion of vaccine-hesitant parents [31]. Providers are in a unique position to help parents opt for HPV vaccination by providing specific, nonjudgmental, and reassuring information. This builds trust and is essential for same-day vaccination. Presenting the HPV vaccine as the default option (and presenting it early and often), being honest about side effects, and focusing on building and maintaining trust can help persuade or turn the tide for parents who have concerns regarding the HPV vaccine. Being prepared to answer common questions regarding the HPV vaccine and providing resources and information also will assist in credibility (see Table 1).

Disclosure

M. Henley has no disclosures of any commercial or financial conflicts of interest or any funding sources related to the topic in this article.

References

[1] Bosch FX, Lorincz A, Muñoz N, et al. The causal relation between human papillomavirus and cervical cancer. J Clin Pathol 2002;55:244–65.

[2] Petrosky E, Bocchini JA Jr, Hariri S, et al. Use of 9-valent human papillomavirus (HPV) vaccine: updated HPV vaccination recommendations of the Advisory Committee on Immunization Practices. MMWR Morb Mortal Wkly Rep 2015;64:300–4.

[3] Centers for Disease Control. Use of 9-valent human papillomavirus (HPV) vaccine: updated HPV vaccination recommendations of the advisory committee on immunization practices. MMWR 2015;64(11):300–4.

[4] Saraiya M, Unger ER, Thompson TD, et al, HPV Typing of Cancers Workgroup. US assessment of HPV types in cancers: implications for current and 9-valent HPV vaccines. J Natl Cancer Inst 2015;107:djv086.

[5] Markowitz LE, Gee J, Chesson H, et al. Ten years of human papillomavirus vaccination in the United States. Acad Pediatr 2018;18(2S):S3–10.

[6] Guo F, Cofie LE, Berenson AB. Cervical cancer incidence in young U. S. females after human papillomavirus vaccine introduction. Am J Prev Med 2018;55(2):197–204.

[7] Bianco A, Mascaro V, Zucco R, et al. Parent perspectives on childhood vaccination: how to deal with vaccine hesitancy and refusal? Vaccine 2019;37:984–90.

[8] Walker TY, Elam-Evans LD, Yankey D, et al. National, regional, state, and selected local area vaccination coverage among adolescents aged 13–17 years — United States, 2018. MMWR Morb Mortal Wkly Rep 2019;68:718–23.

[9] Van Dyne EA, Henley SJ, Saraiya M, et al. Trends in human papillomavirus-associated cancers - United States, 1999 - 2015. MMWR Morb Mortal Wkly Rep 2018;67(33):918–24.

[10] Patel P, Berenson AB. Sources of HPV vaccine hesitancy in parents. Hum Vaccin Immunother 2008;9:2649–53.

[11] Gilkey MB, Calo WA, Marciniak MW, et al. Parents who refuse or delay HPV vaccine: differences in vaccination behavior, beliefs, and clinical communication preferences. Hum Vaccin Immunother 2008;13:680–6.

[12] Karafillakis E, Simas C, Jarrett C, et al. HPV vaccination in a context of public mistrust and uncertainty: a systematic literature review of determinants of HPV vaccine hesitancy in Europe. Hum Vaccin Immunother 2008;15(7–8):1615–27.

[13] Brown B, Gabra MI, Pellman H. Reasons for acceptance or refusal of human papillomavirus vaccine in a California pediatric practice. Papillomavirus Res 2017;3:42–5.

[14] Rosenberg J. Unpacking the root causes and consequences of vaccine hesitancy. Am J Manag Care 2019. In Focus Blog.

[15] Gilkey MB, Calo WA, Moss JL, et al. Provider communication and HPV vaccination: the impact of recommendation quality. Vaccine 2016;34:1187–92.

[16] Shay LA, Baldwin AS, Betts AC, et al. Parent-provider communication of HPV vaccine hesitancy. Pediatrics 2018;141(6):2017–312.

[17] Lo B. HPV vaccine and adolescents' sexual activity. BMJ 2006;332(7550):1106–7.

[18] Donken R, Ogilvie GS, Bettinger JA, et al. Effect of human papillomavirus vaccination on sexual behavior among young females. Can Fam Physician 2018;64(7):509–13.

[19] Bragazzi NL, Barberis I, Rosselli R, et al. How often people google for vaccination: qualitative and quantitative insights from a systematic search of the web-based activities using Google Trends. Hum Vaccin Immunother 2017;13(2):464–9.

[20] Lindley MC, Jeyarajah J, Yankey D, et al. Comparing human papillomavirus vaccine knowledge and intentions among parents of boys and girls. Hum Vaccin Immunother 2016;12(6):1519–27.

[21] Betsch C, Sachse K. Debunking vaccination myths: strong risk negations can increase perceived vaccination risks. Health Psychol 2013;32(2):146–55.

[22] Gilkey MB, Malo TL, Shah PD, et al. Quality of physician communication about human papillomavirus vaccine: findings from a national survey. Cancer Epidemiol Biomarkers Prev 2015;24:1673–9.

[23] Fenton AT, Eun TJ, Clark JA, et al. Indicated or elective? The association of providers' words with HPV vaccine receipt. Hum Vaccin Immunother 2018;14(10):2503–9.

[24] Shen SC, Dubey V. Addressing vaccine hesitancy: clinical guidance for primary care physicians working with parents. Can Fam Physician 2019;65:175–81.

[25] Laranjo L, Arguel A, Neves AL, et al. The influence of social networking sites on health behavior change: a systematic review and meta-analysis. J Am Med Inform Assoc 2015;22:243–56.

[26] Clark SJ, Cowan AE, Filipp SL, et al. Parent perception of provider interactions influences HPV vaccination status of adolescent females. Clin Pediatr (Phila) 2016;55:701–6.

[27] Thompson EL, Rosen BL, Vamos CA, et al. Human papillomavirus vaccination: what are the reasons for nonvaccination among U.S. adolescents? J Adolesc Health 2017;61(3):288–93.

[28] Maglione MA, Das L, Raaen L, et al. Safety of vaccines used for routine immunization of US children: a systematic review. Pediatrics 2014;134(2):325–37.

[29] Arana JE, Harrington T, Cano M, et al. Post-licensure safety monitoring of quadrivalent human papillomavirus vaccine in the Vaccine Adverse Event Reporting System (VAERS), 2009–2015. Vaccine 2018;36(13):1781–8.

[30] Fu LY, Zimet GD, Latkin CA, et al. Associations of trust and healthcare provider advice with HPV vaccine acceptance among African American patients. Vaccine 2017;35(5):802–7.

[31] Benin AL, Wisler-Scher DJ, Colson E, et al. Qualitative analysis of mothers' decision-making about vaccines for infants: the importance of trust. Pediatrics 2006;117(5):1532–41.

[32] Farmar AM, Love-Osborne K, Chicester K, et al. Achieving high adolescent HPV vaccination coverage. Pediatrics 2016;138(5):e20152653.

[33] Centers for Disease Control and Prevention. Genital HPV infection - CDC fact sheet 2012. Available at: www.cdc.gov/std/HPV/STDFact-HPV.htm. Accessed September 1, 2019.

[34] Gowda C, Dempsey AF. The rise (and fall?) of parental vaccine hesitancy. Hum Vaccin Immunother 2013;9(8):1755–62.

[35] Bianco A, Zucco R, Nobile CG, et al. Parental information-seeking behaviour in childhood. Parents seeking health-related information on the Internet: cross-sectional study. J Med Internet Res 2013;15(9):e204.

[36] Nyhan B, Reifler J, Richey S, et al. Effective messages in vaccine promotion: a randomized trial. Pediatrics 2014;133:e835–42.

[37] Gerend MA, Shepherd JE. Using message framing to promote acceptance of the human papillomavirus vaccine. Health Psychol 2007;26:745–52.

[38] Ferguson E, Gallagher L. Message framing with respect to decisions about vaccination: the roles of frame valence, frame method and perceived risk. Br J Psychol 2007;98(Pt 4): 667–80.

[39] Dempsey A. Communicating with families about HPV vaccine. J Clin Outcomes Manag 2017;24(3).

Moving?

Make sure your subscription moves with you!

To notify us of your new address, find your **Clinics Account Number** (located on your mailing label above your name), and contact customer service at:

Email: journalscustomerservice-usa@elsevier.com

800-654-2452 (subscribers in the U.S. & Canada)
314-447-8871 (subscribers outside of the U.S. & Canada)

Fax number: 314-447-8029

Elsevier Health Sciences Division
Subscription Customer Service
3251 Riverport Lane
Maryland Heights, MO 63043

*To ensure uninterrupted delivery of your subscription, please notify us at least 4 weeks in advance of move.

Printed and bound by CPI Group (UK) Ltd, Croydon, CR0 4YY

08/05/2025

01864697-0002